SPINAL MANIPULATION

Spinal Manipulation

J. F. Bourdillon FRCS FRCS (C)

Past President, North American Academy
of Manipulative Medicine
Formerly Consultant Orthopaedic Surgeon to the
Gloucestershire Royal Hospital

Third Edition

William Heinemann Medical Books Limited
London
and
Appleton-Century-Crofts
New York

First published 1970
Second Edition 1973
Revised reprint 1975
Third Edition 1982
Reprinted 1982

© J. F. Bourdillon, 1982

ISBN 0-433-03632-X (U.K.)
ISBN 0-8385-8641-4 (U.S.A.) Author code: A-8641-1

Printed in Great Britain by
The Whitefriars Press Ltd., Tonbridge

Foreword

Osteopathy is an emotive word, especially when mentioned among doctors, or should I say allopaths, yet manipulation must be the oldest form of surgery ever practised. Why has osteopathy gained itself this bad name in many quarters? The author answers this question very clearly and sensibly in his introductory chapter, and as I have known him since we studied medicine together I can vouch both for the facts and for his progress to his present position. His conversion was not at all of the instant type like Saint Paul, but I think it fair comment that the motor-bicycle accident which damaged his own back at Crackington Haven was the initial stepping stone.

As I followed the author's increasing interest and involvement in manipulative surgery I was fascinated with the reaction of a first-class brain with scientific training to the facts as he saw them. John Bourdillon was perhaps most fortunate in also being extremely dexterous and I am sure this has stood him well in his adoption of the techniques he describes here. He has done us a great service in explaining in clear, factual and scientific language much that has been wrapped up as an art in the past and the illustrations in particular are absolutely excellent in this respect.

There is no book which I know of comparable to this one and I feel honoured and a little excited at the prospect of introducing it to others.

Royal Postgraduate Medical School   Selwyn Taylor
Hammersmith Hospital
London W12 OHS
April 1970

Preface to the First Edition

So many people have helped me in my efforts to produce this book that it would be impossible to mention them all.

I must gratefully acknowledge the permission given by the British Medical Journal for the extracts from a 1910 Editorial; from H. K. Lewis & Company Limited to quote from Timbrell Fisher's Treatment by Manipulation; from the J. B. Lippincott Company for permission to quote from an article by Dr. Horace Gray in the International Clinics, and from the Editors of Brain and the Anatomical Record for permission to reproduce the dermatome charts in the papers by Sir Henry Head and by Drs. Keegan and Garrett respectively.

It is invidious to thank individuals but I must express my gratitude for the cheerful and untiring help which I have received from the British Columbia Medical Library Service and from the Staff of the Records Department of the Gloucestershire Royal Hospital.

I cannot leave out my secretary who has typed, typed and retyped every word that is here written, nor indeed, my wife, who has in turn typed, criticised, encouraged and proof read. Finally, it would be very discourteous not to mention both my long suffering model and her husband who took the photographs.

I have endeavoured to shed light on the mystery that surrounds manipulation, to explain how to do it in terms that I hope will be easy enough to understand, to produce a working hypothesis as a basis for argument and a guide for research, and to show some of the reasons why I believe that it is essential that Medicine should incorporate this teaching into its structure.

Vancouver, B.C.   J.F.B.
1970

Preface to the Third Edition

For this edition major changes have been made in the text. Further evidence is presented for the belief that hypertonus in muscle is the basic cause of the pain. New techniques of examination are described, including methods by which the loss of movement can be precisely defined. The non-specific treatment techniques described in earlier editions have been omitted because I believe that they ought no longer to be considered good enough.

The specific techniques are retained with some modifications. They are specific as to level, but not fully so as to direction and are now classed as semi-specific. Fully specific high velocity techniques are described and, in order to use these, precise definition of the movement defect is essential.

A new class of technique is described in which there is no high velocity thrust. First described by Dr. Fred Mitchell (Sen) these use the patient's own muscular effort as the corrective force. The only force used by the manipulator is that required to prevent movement. Dr. Mitchell used the term "muscle energy" but I have preferred "isometric" techniques because this word is already understood by the profession. Because they are more gentle, isometric techniques can be used in patients for whom high velocity thrusting would be unsafe.

My thanks are due to a number of doctors of osteopathy who have been very helpful in instructing me in these new concepts. In particular I want to thank Dr. Paul Kimberly, Dr. Philip Greenman and Dr. Edward Stiles. Dr. Kimberly also very kindly gave permission to use his concept of the resistant barrier and descriptions of techniques from his *Outline of Osteopathic Manipulative Procedures* (published by the Kirksville College of Osteopathic Medicine, Kirksville, Mi., U.S.A.).

Vancouver, B.C.   J.F.B.
1982

Contents

1

Introduction

The art of manipulation of the spine is a very old one. It has been practised since prehistoric times and was known to Hippocrates and to the physicians of ancient Rome.

Bone setters have existed for as long as there are records, and in many countries, including England, they still exist. In the library of the Royal College of Surgeons in London is a book dated 1656 which is a revision by one Robert Turner of a work by an Augustinian monk, Friar Moulton, entitled *The Compleat Bone Setter*.

In 1745 the Surgeons eventually separated from the old City company of Barbers and Surgeons of London and became a new company which, in the early nineteenth century, became the Royal College of Surgeons of England.

Prior to this time it is probable that the bone setters were regarded as the Orthopaedic Surgeons of their day, but for reasons that are unknown they became less and less respectable as the art of medicine and surgery gradually became transformed into a science.

The art of bone setting appears often to have been passed from father to son, and there is some evidence to suggest that an hereditary trait is of some value. Certainly it is accepted experience that some learn the art of manipulation much more easily than others. The art was not at any time supported by adequate scientific investigation, but experience with patients previously handled by bone setters shows that they can sometimes be surprisingly skilful. Unfortunately their explanation to their clients of what they do is often quite unacceptable to the medical profession and reflects their almost total lack of knowledge of anatomy, physiology or pathology.

The advent of routine radiography, the research into the anatomy of the intervertebral joint and of the disc and the operative findings have conclusively shown that there is not "a little bone out of place". The orthodox medical profession has, therefore, found itself unable to accept the manipulator's claims.

1

Unfortunately, the rejection of these claims has provided the profession with a most convenient cloak behind which to hide its jealousy of the manipulator's success and its dislike of anything new and strange. This, however, is a poor excuse for failure to investigate, test and research into the treatment which these practitioners use, even if it were less successful than it is known to be.

It is easy in this modern day to forget that only a few generations ago medicine was an art and the large majority of medical and surgical treatments were based on the results of practical experience rather than on firm scientific foundation.

The reasons for the neglect of research into the art of manipulation are manifold but the results of this neglect are potentially serious to the profession. It has already resulted in the development of two schools of manipulative treatment separate from the profession as well as to the continued prosperity of a multitude of irregular practitioners styling themselves under a variety of names.

The celebrated John Hunter is quoted by Timbrell Fisher[1] as having said, "Nothing can promote contraction of a joint so much as motion before the disease is removed. ... When all inflammation is gone off and healing has begun, a little motion frequently repeated is necessary to prevent healing taking place with the parts fixed in one position." This, unfortunately, was interpreted by Hunter's successors in such a way that they felt justified in allowing adhesions to form in a joint and relying on their ability afterwards to mobilise them.

This treatment is still accepted as being of the greatest value in infective arthritis. Unfortunately the concept was extended to joints stiffened by injury and it is now well known that in such patients early movement of the injured joint is a much more reliable method of restoring function.

It must be remembered that, at that time, there were no x-rays, tuberculosis was common in England and diagnosis presented serious difficulties. The standard of orthodox treatment of joint disease was far from satisfactory, many ending up with a joint excision or amputation. At the same time the fear of litigation against bone setters was almost non-existent and there can be no doubt that patients were injured by forcible manipulation of infected joints.

The famous British surgeon Sir James Paget was one of the few of his day who appreciated the value of manipulative therapy and in his lecture published in the *British Medical Journal*[2] he gave the following advice: "Learn then, to imitate what is good and avoid what is bad in the practice of bone setters ... too long rest is, I believe, by far the most frequent cause of delayed recovery after injuries of joints and not only to injured joints, but to those that are kept at rest because parts near them have been injured."

The medical profession of the time paid little heed to Paget's advice. Hugh Owen Thomas used to teach that an overdose of rest was impossible. This appears to have started at a time when he had a bitter quarrel with his father who, like his grandfather, was a bone setter. He is quoted by Timbrell Fisher[1] as having written a letter in reply to Paget's lecture in which he said, "For many years after the commencement of my experience in surgery I had the opportunity of observing the practice of those who had acquired a good reputation for skill as successful manipulators. ... I cannot find suitable cases on which I would perform the deception known as passive motion."

Later, however, his own suffering led Thomas to visit one of the most celebrated bone setters of the nineteenth century and the following passage in another letter quoted by Timbrell Fisher[1] reflects the change of heart produced by personal experience. "In my own case, after submitting to Mr. Hutton's manipulation, I was instantly relieved of that pain, tension and coldness in the joint that I had suffered for six years, and was able to walk. ... Professional men accounted for the manifest change in my condition on one hypothesis and another, whilst all affected to smile at my ignorance and delusion ... I had been lame and in pain and could now walk and was at ease ... and had the whole College of Surgeons clearly demonstrated to their entire satisfaction that I could not possibly have been benefited by Mr. Hutton's treatment, my opinion would not have been in the smallest degree shaken by it."

One of the difficulties arises from the fact that the symptoms produced by a spinal joint derangement can be surprisingly diverse and are often manifest at a distance from the spine rather than in the spine itself. Another arises from the anatomy, the spinal joint being deeply placed under cover of powerful muscles so that it is only indirectly available to the examining finger. A possible third is that the art of successful spinal manipulation comes much more easily to some people than to others, although the reasons for this are not understood.

Another factor in the neglect of this branch of work by the medical profession has been the claims made by manipulators in which they said they were able to cure all manner of diseases by manipulation of the spine. This claim was so obviously unacceptable that it tended to blind the medical profession to what the manipulators were really doing. The reasons for this claim, and a possible explanation of it, are discussed in a later chapter. The effect of these extravagant claims was so to alienate the medical profession, that they were unprepared to accept anything which the manipulators said, nor were they even prepared to believe the patients who said they had benefited.

The general public is notorious for pursuing the unorthodox even when experience later shows the stupidity of this action. In the case of the manipulators however, experience showed that the public could get genuine relief from the symptoms of spinal derangements by their treatment and this natural tendency was greatly reinforced. Because of this public demand, irregular practitioners have persisted and increased in numbers.

In the last 100 years two major schools of manipulative therapy have developed and their practitioners are now widespread through many parts of the world. In spite of this, there are still large numbers of practising "natural" manipulators, the successors to the old bone setters, and some of these may still be found without basic scientific training of any kind.

From time to time the voices of highly respected and competent doctors of medicine have been raised in favour of manipulative treatment, but until after the 1939–45 war, the number of such medical manipulators was small and they were generally despised by their colleagues.

In my student days, in the University of Oxford, a special meeting of the Medical Society (the Osler Society) was called and all medical students were specially requested to attend even if not members of the Society. The meeting was addressed by one of the most famous physicians of the age in a deliberate attempt to brainwash his hearers against manipulators, although at that time I did not understand this. It was interesting later to reflect that some of the things which he said displayed his total ignorance of the subject.

There always has been evidence available that patients have felt that they had been materially helped by manipulators and it seems therefore to be a pity that their work should be openly and viciously condemned without even being investigated. Unfortunately, this type of criticism is only too common today.

After leaving Oxford University my subsequent training was at St. Thomas's Hospital where manipulative treatment was practised at that time by Dr. James Mennell in the physiotherapy department. By this time, however, it was already my intention to enter the field of orthopaedic surgery and I was strongly advised by the orthopaedic surgeons to have nothing to do with his department. Even within his own hospital he, and later his successor Dr. James Cyriax, were considered to be little better than outcasts.

The two modern manipulative schools are undoubtedly successors to the old bone setters in spite of their claims to have been started *ab initio* by their respective founders. The first of these was the osteopathic school which was founded by Andrew Taylor Still (1828–1917). Still was registered as a medical practitioner in Missouri, but some doubt has been cast on the quality of his training. According to Northup,[9] he entered Kansas City College of Physicians and Surgeons but, with the advent of the Civil War, dropped out of the course in order to enlist. His name does not appear in the catalogue of 1891 which lists the Kansas City College graduates up to that year. It appears that his training was completed by preceptorship as, indeed, was that of most physicians in the United States at that time. Hildreth[10] reproduces a certificate of registration in Adair county in 1883 and another certificate dated 1893 which states that Still was on the roll of physicians and surgeons in Macon County as early as 1874.

According to Gevitz[11], Still's education was partly at his father's side and from texts in anatomy, physiology and materia medica. At that time medical treatment tended to be brutal and Still became very dissatisfied. He had already started to question the validity of the orthodox teaching before three of his family died of cerebrospinal meningitis in 1864 in spite of the best efforts of a fellow practitioner.

In about 1880 Still's ideas began to crystallise after his experience with a woman who came complaining of shoulder pain. He mobilized the spine and rib joints which relieved her pain but she came back later to tell him that it had also stopped the asthma from which she had suffered for a long time.

The American School of Osteopathy was founded by Still in 1892 and it is of interest that he was at that time registered as a physician. Gevitz suggests that in the early years at the school the training was not what would now be considered adequate.

According to Downing[3], Still's interest started from a personal observation. He is said to have obtained relief from a severe headache by lying on his back with the upper neck supported by a rope slung between two trees.

Unfortunately, he antagonised the profession of his day by his attitude to them, by his shrewd business instinct and his claims to cure all manner of disease.

The osteopathic profession in the United States has, during this century, made great strides forward. D.O.'s are now equally licensed with M.D.'s throughout the U.S.A. and are trained in surgery of all kinds as well as in other specialties. Unfortunately, osteopathic colleges in other countries have not all achieved the same standard.

The second manipulative school is that of chiropractic, which was started in 1895 in Davenport, Iowa, U.S.A. by D. D. Palmer who is described as a "self-educated erstwhile grocer" in a book on chiropractic published in 1962.[4]

The start of chiropractic is said to date from a specific incident when Palmer manipulated the thoracic vertebrae of a negro porter and by this means cured him of deafness from which he had suffered for some years. On the face of it, this is a fantastic and totally unacceptable claim. In a later chapter, however, the author records his own experience in which the function of the inner ear was apparently significantly altered by a manipulation at this level. For the present argument, the fact that Palmer claims at that time to have manipulated a specific vertebra indicates at least a modicum of knowledge and experience of manipulative treatment. That incident is considered to be the starting point of chiropractic but it is clear that Palmer must have been working on his ideas for some years before. It seems likely that he actually learned techniques from some other person, either a bone setter or an osteopath.

Like osteopathy, the art of chiropractic has spread far and wide, particularly in North America. This has happened in spite of the fact that even the more modern books on chiropractic contain passages which are nonsense to those grounded in the basic sciences of orthodox medicine. Indeed, in some parts of North America it appears that their relative popularity with the public is at least partly due to the fact that they are still not accepted by the profession at large whereas, with its research and development, osteopathy has become more respectable.

It is well known that it is impossible to "fool all the people all the time" and there is no doubt that a significant proportion of those who go to chiropractors for treatment, receive benefit. The fact that their theories are unacceptable must not be allowed to blind the profession to this. It should, rather, be regarded as a challenge to the profession to develop adequate theories that will explain their successes and better methods of achieving this success.

Industrial injuries in Canada are handled very largely by a nation-wide organisation of Workmen's Compensation Boards. One of the major problems which these Boards have to handle is the large numbers of industrial injuries to the back. The results of orthodox treatment of these injuries has proved to be far from satisfactory, and at the present time, at least in the province of British Columbia, the Compensation Board has authority to pay for chiropractic treatment for such people should they elect to have this rather than treatment from a medical practitioner. A claimant may also elect to change from a medical practitioner to a chiropractor for treatment, if his general practitioner agrees and, in this case also, the Workmen's Compensation Board will pay for chiropractic treatment up to a certain maximum. The prepaid medical insurance plans also have a clause in their contract accepting responsibility for chiropractors' accounts up to a fixed annual figure.

The attitude of the orthodox medical profession to anything strange and new has often been far from helpful and far from scientific. An editorial in the *British Medical Journal* in 1910[5] reads:

"In the sphere of medicine there is a vast area of 'undeveloped land' which Mr. Lloyd George has somehow failed to include in his Budget. It comprises many methods of treatment which are scarcely taught at all in the schools, which find no place in textbooks and which consequently the 'superior person' passes with gown uplifted to avoid a touch that is deemed pollution. The superior person is, as has more than once been pointed out, one of the greatest obstacles to progress.

"Rational medicine should take as its motto Molière's saying 'Je prends mon bien ou je le trouve'; whatever can be used as a weapon in this warfare against disease belongs to it of right. . . . Now Dr. Bryce has witnessed the mysteries of osteopathy and tells us what he saw in a paper published in this week's issue. . . . The results, recorded by him are of themselves sufficient to justify us in calling attention to the method.

"Not to go so far back as Harvey, who was denounced by the leaders of the profession in his day as a circulator or quack, we need only recall how the open-air treatment of consumption was ridiculed when the idea was first put forward by Bebbington

... famous physicians refused to listen to Pasteur because he was not a medical man; Lister was scoffed at; the laryngoscope was sneered at as a physiological toy; the early ovariotomists in this country were threatened by colleagues with the coroner's court; electricity was looked upon with suspicion; massage, within one's own memory, was regarded as an unclean thing. But even now, the vast field of physiotherapy is largely left to laymen for exploitation."

In an address to the Pacific Interurban Clinical Club Dr. Horace Gray[6] quoted Sir Robert Jones, nephew of Hugh Owen Thomas, "forcible manipulation is a branch of surgery that from time immemorial has been neglected by our profession, and, as a direct consequence, much of it has fallen into the hands of the unqualified practitioner. Let there be no mistake; this has seriously undermined the public confidence, which has on occasion, amounted to open hostility. If we honestly face the facts this attitude should cause us no surprise. No excuse will avail us when a stiff joint, which has been treated for many months by various surgeons and practitioners without effect, rapidly regains its mobility and function at the hands of an irregular practitioner. We should be self-critical and ask why we missed such an opportunity ourselves. The problem is not solved by pointing out mistakes made by the unqualified, the question at issue is their success. Reputations are not made in any walk of life simply by failures. Failures are common to us all and it is a far wiser and more dignified attitude on our part to improve our armamentarium than dwell upon the mistakes made by others."

As the result of representations by osteopaths wishing to obtain official licence in Great Britain, a Select Committee of the House of Lords prepared a report in 1935. Grave deficiencies were shown up in the practice of so-called osteopaths at that time and the Bill to recommend licensing was withdrawn by its sponsors. Recognition has still not been granted in spite of further attempts.

Timbrell Fisher[1] sums up a chapter in which he severely, but justly, criticises the osteopathic profession in England at that time. "Space will not permit the dismal recital of some of the tragedies resulting from this method of treatment that have been observed. Yet it must be admitted that osteopaths sometimes effect cures in patients whose conditions have defied more traditional methods and it is of the utmost importance that we should face this fact squarely and endeavour to ascertain how these cures are brought about. These cases can be classified into three main categories, all of which in reality belong to the domain of manipulative treatment proper.

"In the first category are the patients whose symptoms are actually situated in the spinal column or back and in which the alleviation or cure is due to the breaking down of adhesions in ligament, muscle or aponeurosis.

"In the second category, are the patients whose symptoms are not actually in the spine, but elsewhere, these symptoms being principally in the nature of a neurosis. . . . The simplicity of the theory, the conviction with which it is uttered and the actual treatment by spinal manipulation all act by powerful suggestion. Thus the osteopath may bring about a striking success although his explanation of its occurrence is erroneous.

"In the third category are the patients suffering from pains, often of a neuralgic nature, in various areas of the trunk or limbs. These are referred along with the distribution of the spinal nerves owing to some pressure at their vertebral exits, often due to rheumatism or to the after-effects of injury. Familiar examples include many cases of occipital neuralgia due to pressure upon the upper cervical nerve roots, some cases of brachial or intercostal neuritis causing pain in the extremities or chest, certain cases of obscure abdominal pain often wrongly diagnosed as due to some intra-abdominal lesion and many cases of sciatica due to pressure at the vertebral exits of the spinal nerve roots. Very many cases of such sciatic pain are caused by compression of the sciatic nerve roots by scar tissue due to early vertebral arthritis in the lumbar or lumbo-sacral regions. For many years, the author has practised manipulations of the lumbar spine in this type of case, and, in his experience, the results are usually better than the orthodox immobilisation. . . .

"The osteopaths have also evolved the technique of manipulating the spine and of producing the maximum degree of movement between the individual vertebrae which is worthy of study. . . . As we have already seen the treatment of these conditions really belongs to the realm of manipulative treatment proper, and the danger of building up a revolutionary system of medicine upon such a slender hypothesis, unsupported by scientific evidence, is so incalculable that it is our duty, as guardians of the public health, to fight against this menace."

In England because the osteopaths have not been licensed, the position which they occupy in the eyes of the profession is similar to that which the chiropractors have in Canada. In

North America osteopaths have, for many years, been licensed, permitted to prescribe drugs, perform surgery, run hospitals, sign death certificates and do many of the other official duties which in England are only carried out by the medical profession proper. The fact that many osteopaths and chiropractors in England show clear evidence of continuing success and that the same is true of the unlicensed chiropractors in North America, must be accepted as a considerable challenge to the profession. Without at least a reasonable proportion of success, even the gullibility of the public would not ensure prosperity.

Since the days of the House of Lords Select Committee in 1935, the osteopathic profession in England has gone a long way to put its house in order, both from the point of view of ethics and from the point of view of sound scientific anatomy, physiology and pathology. A considerable mass of research has been done by the various schools of osteopathy, chiefly in the United States but, unfortunately, much of this work requires the confirmation of properly conducted experiments in other centres and it would be nice to see this done from within the medical profession.

The chiropractic school has not yet achieved such a firm scientific foundation and even in recent writings, theories are restated and claims made which are difficult or impossible to reconcile with what the medical profession reasonably considers to be established fact. In spite of this, many chiropractors have obtained, by training and experience, a sufficient knowledge of the vertebral column to be able to make a reasonable assessment of patients, to be aware of the major contra-indications to manipulative therapy and to be able to perform manipulations in such a way that the patients are relieved. They still have a long way to go before they can reasonably be offered the degree of Doctor of Medicine, as has recently been done for the osteopaths in some of the United States.

The existence at the present time in this field of three divergent schools of healing (in addition to others not specifically considered here) must be a source of concern to the medical profession. The orthodox profession is, without doubt, grounded on a very solid scientific foundation and must take pride of place. This fact does not exclude the possibility that the other schools may have something to offer and it is no less unreasonable to condemn them without further investigation than was the condemnation of Lister, Pasteur and so many others who introduced new ideas.

Unfortunately, our orthodox training tends to make us judge anything new by our existing practice and teaching, rather than by going back to basic anatomy, physiology and pathology and it is always difficult to divest oneself of preconceived ideas.

The very success of the osteopaths and the chiropractors should be a stimulus to the orthodox medical profession to undertake an unbiased assessment of their ideas, methods and claims by those competent to do so. In this way alone can their merits be assessed and their good points incorporated into the teaching of medicine as a whole. So far most such investigations have been conducted in a thoroughly unscientific manner and started with a strong bias against the subject under investigation.

With the aid of modern diagnostic tools including x-ray cinematography and electromyography it ought to be possible to elucidate some of the basic problems which still remain unanswered in this field. Such research will, of course, require the expenditure of considerable sums of money and should be conducted in an area where independent observers can assess the effectiveness of both orthodox and unorthodox treatment given to patients in sufficient numbers to allow satisfactory analysis.

The medical profession claims that the healing art is its own exclusive province but unfortunately, the general public does not agree. There will always be the "odd man out" who will tend to seek treatment from an unorthodox practitioner for reasons that are often quite inadequate, but the present position is that many of the public can obtain relief from unorthodox practitioners of manipulative therapy when they do not get the same relief from the orthodox profession.

It is somewhat unexpected to find a man trained as an orthodox orthopaedic surgeon writing as a protagonist of manipulative therapy of this kind and a brief explanation is appropriate. In the interest of clarity and brevity, the first person will be used.

My early interest in the subject was stimulated by a series of coincidences which led to an appreciation of its importance in spite of the early brainwashing to which I have already alluded.

While still a preclinical student I sustained a severe strain of my lumbar spine as a result of a motor-cycle accident. From this I continued to suffer symptoms almost continuously for a number of years and at intervals ever since. I was treated initially, first by one and then by a second very well-known orthopaedic surgeon but the treatments which I received had no effect whatever on the condition other than to give me temporary relief at the time of administration of heat and massage. I well remember the black looks I used to get from the ward sister on teaching rounds in St. Thomas's Hospital in the days when Dame Lloyd Still was matron. When I stood for more than ten minutes at a time my back began to ache so badly that I found it necessary to rest my buttocks on some sort of support and the neighbouring bed was by far the easiest. This disarranged the bed cover and was the cause of the sister's displeasure!

During my war service with the Royal Air Force, I was well grounded in the treatment of acute trauma but the chronic back condition was comparatively rare and my introduction to these in quantity came after my return as Senior Registrar to St. Thomas's Hospital where I quickly learned the then new operation of removal of the protruded intervertebral disc.

At first it seemed that this might be the answer to the problem, but disillusionment very quickly followed in the wake of the negative exploration and unsatisfactory post-operative results. Like many others, I had originally been taught that manipulation under general anaesthetic of the spine of a patient with backache was dangerous and the more so if there was a co-existent sciatica. In my case, the teaching resulted from the unfortunate experience of two of my tutors, in which the manipulation under anaesthetic of the spine of a doctor's wife produced a permanent cauda equina paralysis.

I completed my Registrar training in Cambridge where I learned from R. W. Butler his technique of manipulating spines under general anaesthetic with good results and without any accidents. Working for him I naturally observed and followed his techniques, often with a very satisfactory measure of success. One of the basic points which he taught was a strict avoidance of forced flexion of the spine. The manipulation consisted of traction, rotation and extension only.

I had the good fortune to be called to see a woman with a recurrence of old back trouble. She described how her general practitioner relieved her by a simple manipulation and explained to me how he did it. The movement was similar to one which I had been using under anaesthesia but was accomplished easily and almost without pain. She obtained immediate relief and only required one treatment. Later I discovered the necessity of repeated treatment in many cases in order to give lasting relief.

By this time I was using techniques similar to those used by Butler but without anaesthesia because I had found it to be unnecessary and because of the need for repeated treatment. I have now come to believe that the use of anaesthesia is a great mistake unless in very exceptional circumstances. The intense muscle spasm over destructive lesions is a very valuable ally because it prevents damage being done even if one is unfortunate enough to misdiagnose such a lesion in the early stages and manipulate it. Anaesthesia will of course abolish the protective spasm.

When I first started manipulating spines I was doing so solely for problems in the back itself. I quickly began to find that I was relieving pain in the arms or legs at the same time, even when the symptomatology had not been such as to make me feel that the pain was a referred one. (This will also be discussed in a later chapter.)

My interest in the other schools of manipulative therapy was stimulated by a number of patients whose backs I had manipulated without success, who were kind enough to let me know that subsequent visits to non-medically qualified manipulators had given satisfactory relief. This naturally made me wish to study the methods used by these practitioners. The rules of the profession made it somewhat difficult until by chance I met the late Dr. Donald Turner, then a general practitioner in Folkestone, who himself had learnt the techniques after being relieved of a severe sciatica by an osteopath. He was kind enough to teach me what he knew and from this and from other medical manipulators, I have developed the system which I now use and which I have tried to describe in the chapters on specific joint manipulation which follow.

One of the patients whom Dr. Turner relieved was a woman whose low lumbar spine I had explored on two occasions and from whom I had removed disc protrusions at both the lumbosacral joint and the L4–5 joint. In spite of this she was still crippled by severe symptoms. He succeeded in relieving her and I continued to treat her for many years afterwards when she had recurrences. The main trouble in her case was a sciatic radiation of pain caused by a sacro-iliac strain and I well remember my blank feeling of disbelief when Dr. Turner suggested this possibility. "How," I said to myself, "can the sacro-iliac joint possibly cause a sciatica when there is no conceivable means by which any of the nerves of the sacral plexus can be pressed on by such a joint strain?" Dr. Turner's results and my subsequent experience have, for me, completely proved that a sacro-iliac strain can be the cause of a sciatica, but the precise means by which this pain reference is produced remains a matter of theory for which adequate experimental proof is still lacking.

There are, of course, two joints in the spine which have no intervertebral disc, namely the atlanto-occipital and that between the 1st and 2nd cervical vertebrae. As the result of practical experience I am also satisfied that joint derangements of both the atlanto-occipital and the atlanto-axial joints can cause pain both locally and referred. These findings in the atlanto-occipital, atlanto-axial and sacro-iliac joints strongly suggest that the disc itself is not the only important source of symptoms and possibly not even the most important.

Many authors have arrived by similar means at similar conclusions and have developed theories of their own. My own theories and the reasons for them will be discussed in a later chapter, but for the moment the manipulative techniques will be described on the basis that one is trying to put a stiffened joint through a range of movement, rather than anything more complicated.

Stiffness of the involved joints can be demonstrated both clinically and radiologically. The radiological demonstration requires a comparison of films taken in flexion and extension and, by this, it is possible to determine which joints are not moving at all and which have restricted motion. A knowledge of the normal range in the various joints and of the variations to be considered normal is, of course, essential.

The clinical demonstration depends on the appreciation of movement and of tension differences in the interspinous ligaments. These are more readily felt when the fingers have had considerable experience and this often makes the demonstration somewhat unconvincing to the newcomer.

Some patients are very much easier to examine in this way than others. Severe obesity can make the examination very difficult but unfortunately, there is another group that is equally difficult. These are those people whose subcutaneous tissue is dense and fibrosed so that it feels tough even when they are not unduly obese.

The precise techniques are described later.

The techniques which I use are by no means new. Many of them were, in fact, described by Dr. Thomas Marlin in 1934.[7] At that time he was in charge of what later became the physiotherapy department at University College Hospital, London, and he described in his introduction how he studied osteopathy at one of the colleges in the United States of America. He did this after finding that some of his patients had been relieved by manipulators even when he had failed to help them. He concludes in his introduction, "The day is past when this form of treatment should be regarded as outside the scope of medical practitioners and this book is an attempt to present in readable form, some of those manipulations which I have learned."

He also records that after a demonstration of some of these techniques one of his senior colleagues told him that some of them had been practised in England as long as forty years before his demonstration.

Finally, a word of warning, issued by Mennell.[8] "A simple locking of any of the joints may frequently be relieved by manipulation without an anaesthetic though it is by no means everyone who is able to learn the requisite techniques. . . . It is desirable that the people who fail to acquire the art of manipulation, however competent they may be otherwise, should realise their limitations and leave this branch of the work alone."

REFERENCES

1 Timbrell Fisher, A. G. (1948), *Treatment by Manipulation*, 5th Ed., London, Lewis.
2 Paget, Sir James (1867), Cases that bone setters cure, *Brit. Med. J.* 1, 1–4.
3 Downing, C. H. (1935), *Osteopathic Principles in Disease*, San Francisco, Orozco.
4 Homewood, A. E. (1962), *The Neurodynamics of Vertebral Subluxation*, Publisher unstated.
5 Editorial (1910), *Brit. Med. J.* 2, 638.
6 Gray, H. (1938), Sacro-iliac joint pain, *Int. Clin.* 2, 54–96.
7 Marlin, J. (1934), *Manipulative Treatment*, London, Arnold.
8 Mennell, James (1945), *Treatment by Movement and Massage*, 5th Ed., London, Churchill.
9 Northup, G. W., D.O. (1966), *Osteopathic Medicine. An American Reformation*. American Osteopathic Association, Chicago, Illinois.
10 Hildreth, A. G., D.O. (1938), *The Lengthening Shadow of Dr. Andrew Taylor Still*. Hildreth, Macon, Missouri.
11 Gevitz, Norman, *The D.O.'s, A social history of Osteopathic Medicine*. Ph.D. Dissertation University of Chicago, 1979. Awaiting publication.

2

Anatomy

All doctors in their training acquire a basic working knowledge of the anatomy of the spinal column. The object of this chapter is to refresh the reader's memory on points that he may have forgotten, to go into detail about specific points which are often neglected and to present some evidence suggesting that in certain aspects the standard anatomical teaching is not fully in accord with recent research work.

It is the clinical experience of countless manipulators that patients obtain relief from certain symptoms after manipulation, not only of spinal joints themselves, but of the sacro-iliac joints and, although this is perhaps not so commonly accepted, also of the costovertebral joints. In trying to understand the reasons for the success of manipulation, it is of fundamental importance that one should have an accurate picture of the structure and normal function of the joint concerned.

The classical paper of Mixter and Barr[1] stimulated the interest of the profession in the structure of the intervertebral joint. Since that time, many papers have been published and a great deal of fundamental research has been carried out. Even so, it is important to remember the work that had gone before and an excellent review of this work is given by Armstrong[2] in his introduction.

The Sacro-Iliac Joint

In spite of much recent work on the subject by anatomists, there remains in the minds of many doctors, the idea that this joint is one in which no movement normally takes place. In many old editions of Gray's Anatomy, the joint is described as a diarthrodial joint but with the cartilage plates in close contact and partly united by patches of soft fibro-cartilage and fine interosseous fibres.

Brooke[3] reported the results of examination of 200 sacro-iliac joints. He refers to the articular surface of the sacrum as being "flatly concaved from side to side, the concavity being most

16

marked at the angle between the two limbs. Here the junction between the posterior and upper borders forms a prominent lip which fits into the corresponding depression behind the convex articular surface of the ilium. This constitutes an important interlocking mechanism around which rotation takes place."

Brooke continues to describe the movement which he says is slight but quite definite, both of a gliding and rotatory nature. The gliding can be upwards, downwards, or backwards but the more important movement is rotatory and takes place around the interlocking mechanism of the middle segment which he described.

Brooke went on to say that in the infant and the pregnant woman the joint takes part in the movements of the lower spine but he was unable, in his dissections, to find proof that it also occurs in non-pregnant adults.

With regard to the soft fibro-cartilage and interosseous fibres described in the older editions of Gray's Anatomy, he says, "Certainly in younger subjects of both sexes, the joint surfaces are quite smooth and separate and the presence of congenital fibrous strands bridging across the joint described by Henri Vignes must be an extremely rare condition." He concludes with the summary, "The old description that the joint was an amphiarthrosis, was the description of a pathological change. The normal joint is of the diarthrodial type and in all probability takes part in movements backwards and forwards of the lumbar spine.

"The joint cavity itself is well defined with a continuous fringe of synovial membrane and, at times, the addition of an accessory limb. It is a diarthrodial joint, resembling in every characteristic any other joint of this type, becoming amphiarthrodial only under certain pathological conditions."

In 1936 Pitkin and Pheasant published a series of papers on Sacroarthrogenic Telalgia.[4] This term they coin to describe "a syndrome of pain which originates in the sacro-iliac and sacrolumbar articulations and accessory ligaments. The referred pain affects gluteal and/or sacral regions and may affect any part or all parts of the lower extremities except the internal crural and plantar regions."

They conclude:

1 That sacro-iliac mobility can be demonstrated in vivo by measuring the movements of the ilia;
2 That in the standing position all motions of the trunk, with

the exception of flexion and extension, are normally associated with unpaired antagonistic movements of the ilia about a transverse axis that passes through the centre of the symphysis pubis;

3 That rotation and lateral bending of the sacrum do not normally occur alone, but as correlated motions that are coincidental to antagonistic movements of the ilia.

They also state in their conclusions that Sacrarthrogenic Telalgia is not the result of irritation or compression of the trunks of peripheral nerves and secondly, that abnormal sacro-iliac mobility is a potent cause of abnormal ligament tension that produces this syndrome.

Horace Gray[5] discusses the detailed anatomy of the sacro-iliac joint with a summary of the evidence for the existence of mobility. Describing both forward and backward torsion of the ilium on the sacrum, he expresses the opinion that "matching lumps and hollows need move only one millimeter and stick at the limit of normal motion to cause pain; and that this working hypothesis fits as well as any other hitherto offered to explain the clinical observation of pain in the back relieved abruptly by manipulation without anaesthetic."

In the tenth edition of Cunningham's Textbook of Anatomy[6] the joint is described as a synovial joint but the surfaces are often irregular, causing a certain amount of interlocking between the facets. Movement is described as being greatly restricted by the irregularity of the articular facets and the thickness and disposition of the dorsal sacro-iliac ligaments.

Weisl[7] investigated the movements of the sacro-iliac joint by radiographic methods in the living subject. The pelvis was fixed in a special apparatus which also located the x-ray tube and cassette so as to produce comparable pictures. The position of the subject was then altered by various degrees of flexion and extension of the trunk and legs. He reports the following findings:

"In a minority of subjects the sacral displacement was such that the sacral line remained parallel to its position at rest. Angular displacement occurred much more frequently and it was possible to locate an axis of rotation. It was situated approximately 10 cm below the promontory in the normal subjects, both recumbent and standing, and was placed a little higher in puerperal women. Contrary to the belief of previous authors, the site of this axis was variable and in a majority of subjects, either the axis moved more than 5 cm following various changes of posture, or angular and parallel movement of the sacrum occurred in the same subject. . . .

"The position of this axis of rotation differed from that described by earlier authors who based their opinions only on the examination of the sacro-iliac articular surfaces. . . ."

He also found that by these means there was no difference in the range of movement between males and females except in the puerperal state and that difference in the range of movement could not be correlated with the height, weight or sacral curve index in the individual. The maximum constant movement was a ventral movement of the promontory of 5.6 $\pm$ 1.4 mm in the change of position from recumbency to standing. The movements on flexion and extension of the trunk were of smaller range and less consistent.

In recent editions of Gray's Anatomy[8] the sacro-iliac joint is described as being a synovial joint and, in the adult, it is marked by a number of "irregular elevations and depressions. These irregularities, which are more pronounced in the male, fit into one another and provide a locking device restricting movement and contributing to the stability of the sacro-iliac joint. . . . In the elderly, it is usual to find that the joint cavity is at least partly obliterated by the presence of fibrous or fibro-cartilaginous adhesions and synostosis may occur. These changes are more common in the male."

On applied anatomy, Gray describes the occurrence of sacro-iliac strain with locking of the joints in the abnormal position, requiring forcible manipulation for its reduction. This is mentioned in connection with relaxation of the pelvic ligaments occurring in pregnancy.

There are striking differences in the conclusions drawn by Brooke, by Pitkin and Pheasant and by Weisl from their studies of the sacro-iliac joint. The chief difference is in the location of the centre of movement of the joint and the findings are so far at variance as to suggest that, by the nature of their observations, one observer saw and measured one type of movement and another saw evidence of movement of a different type occurring at the same joint.

From the clinical point of view, the most important movement of the sacro-iliac joint is one which may well have been excluded by the technique used by Weisl in his experiments. This is the antagonistic movement about a transverse axis through the symphysis pubis described by Pitkin and Pheasant. This movement cannot occur without producing torsion of the pelvis involving rotation of the ilia on the sacrum in opposite directions. Brooke[3] actually concluded that such torsional movements occur in the normal act of walking. Such rotations of ilium on sacrum could well occur around the interlocking mechanism of the middle segment described by Brooke. As a result of the innominate rotation the sacrum twists about its long axis so that the auricular surface faces more posteriorly on the side on which the innominate rotates with the iliac crest becoming more posterior. The auricular surface of the sacrum on the same side is also tilted to face more caudally because of a small amount of rotation of the sacrum about an antero-posterior axis. This alteration of the position of the sacrum is, of course, transmitted to the superincumbent spine.

Fryette[13] points out that there are many anatomical variations in the sacrum. In particular he shows photographs of what he describes as the three main types.

Type A has the typical shape of the first segment. The dorsal transverse measurement is slightly greater than the ventral. This he finds is associated commonly with transverse (thoracic type) lumbosacral facet joints.

Type B has the dorsal transverse measurement of the first segment smaller than the ventral. The associated facets are sagittal (lumbar type).

Type C has one articular surface sloping out and the other in. In other words one half of the sacrum is like Type A and the other half like Type B with the corresponding facet joint alignments.

These observations suggest a further reason why pelvic joint dysfunction does not always follow a standard pattern.

The function of the three joints in the pelvic ring is probably the least well understood of any in the body. There is now no room for doubt that the sacro-iliac joints are mobile, diarthrodial joints although they have only a small range of movement. In the normal the symphysis pubis permits only twisting between the pubic bones. In the abnormal, however, other movements may occur including translation (upward on one side, downward on the other) and separation. This translation can indeed sometimes be seen in the x-ray. (Fig. 14) See Kapandji[9] for an analysis of the effect of posture on the joints of the pelvis.

Rotation at the sacro-iliac joint causing forward displacement of the pubic bones at the symphysis on the side upon which the individual is bearing his weight in standing was demonstrated by Schunke[10].

The movement of the sacrum between the ilia is complex, the sacrum may rock in flexion and extension between the ilia or it may twist. The complexities and the combinations which are found clinically defy any simple mechanical explanation. While this difficulty at first bothers anyone who thinks about it, it is not really so surprising. Evidence will be mentioned later which shows that the problem with which we are primarily concerned is abnormal tension in muscle. It is not the fact that the joint is prevented from moving properly so much as that one, or more, muscles are in a state of abnormal tension. The object of the treatment therefore, is to obtain relaxation of the muscle or muscles concerned. The movements needed to do this need not necessarily fit into a mechanical model which omits consideration of muscle function.

Pelvic torsion produces an apparent inequality in the length of the legs and seriously affects the accuracy of the ordinary clinical methods of estimating any difference in leg length.

It will readily be appreciated that if the pelvis is in a state of torsion, the anterior superior spine on one side will be higher than on the other and any measurement taken from this point for the purpose of estimating relative leg length, will be falsified by the difference in level.

Methods of estimating differences in leg length are described and discussed in the chapter on examination.

The sacro-iliac joints lie posterior to the coronal plane passing through the centre of the hip joints. If, therefore, there is a state of pelvic torsion, with the left innominate rotated backwards relative to the sacrum, the distance on the left side from the uppermost part of the sacral ala to the heel is reduced.

This alteration in effective leg length by movement of the sacro-iliac joint is illustrated in Fig. 1. With the subject erect an alteration in the angular position of the sacro-iliac joint will cause an alteration in the angle made by a fixed line on the innominate bone with the horizontal (the only alternative would be tilting of the spine forwards or backward out of the erect posture). This alteration in the tilt of the innominate bone will, of course, produce a change in the angle θ. This is the angle between a vertical dropped from the centre of movement of the hip joint and a line joining that centre of movement to a fixed part of the sacro-iliac joint. The position of the centre of movement as described by Brooke is used for convenience. Simple geometry shows that when the angle θ is reduced, the distance between the floor and the fixed point in the sacro-iliac

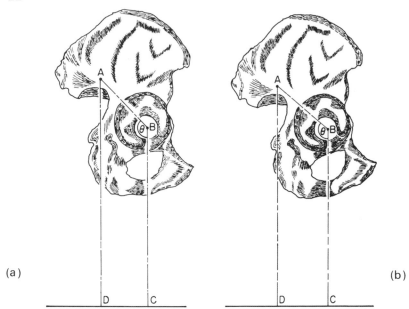

Fig. 1 (a) Innominate in the anterior position. (b) Innominate in the posterior position. The line B—C remains the same length but A—D has become shorter.

joint is also reduced, producing an apparent shortening of the limb.

Differences in the actual leg length of the lower limb are common. In the majority the differences are minor, being less than a quarter of an inch. Differences in length of more than a quarter of an inch are not uncommon and can, of course, result from malunion of fractures or from other pathological changes in the lower limbs. Leg inequality is sometimes familial and in these the difference may well be half an inch or more.

In patients with leg inequality there is a natural tendency for the pelvis to adopt the twisted position which most nearly levels the antero-superior surface of the sacrum. This means that on the side of the longer leg, the sacro-iliac joint will habitually adopt a posture with the innominate rotated posteriorly with respect to the sacrum. Unfortunately, the stresses and strains of life tend to cause the sacro-iliac joint to stiffen in that position, the more so if the subject is engaged in a heavy occupation. Simple stiffness of the sacro-iliac joint is not necessarily a cause of symptoms but it can easily become so and an example of a patient who has suffered from acute low back pain due to a sacro-iliac strain is given in the Appendix (Case 1). In this particular instance, the sacro-iliac strain was caused by the prolonged wearing of an artificial limb which was one inch too long.

In a person with an actual difference in the length of the lower limb, the adoption by the pelvis of the twisted position will diminish the tilting of the sacrum. Unfortunately, the backward movement of the innominate on one side and the forward movement on the other causes a rotation of the sacrum about its long axis. This rotation is of course, transmitted to the lumbar spine. It seems probable that there is a righting mechanism which tends to correct the rotation in the lumbar spine in order to preserve the forward pointing attitude of the head. This twist and the corrective forces which it causes, unfortunately tend to predispose the patient to trouble in the lumbar region and sometimes even higher. For this reason, observation of leg length difference is most important in patients complaining of back symptoms. If a difference is found in excess of a quarter inch, a correction by means of an alteration to the shoe is frequently necessary. If the leg length difference continues unobserved and uncorrected, the constant (if minor) strain which it produces, may make it difficult or impossible to cure the lumbar symptoms.

If a fixed pelvic torsion occurs as a result of an injury in a patient with equal legs, the effect on the lumbar spine is essentially similar. The rotatory displacement of the sacrum about its long axis is the same, but there is now a tilting of that long axis towards the side on which the innominate is in the posterior position. In a case of leg length difference where the difference is too great to be fully corrected by the pelvic torsion, the tilt of the sacral long axis is of course in the opposite direction. In either case, recognition and treatment of the sacro-iliac strain may be of vital importance in the care of the patient.

In this connection it may be worth restating the author's feeling of blank disbelief at the first mention of the sacro-iliac joint as a cause of back and leg pain. This disbelief arose from the idea popular at that time that referred leg pain was caused by actual pressure on nerves or nerve roots.

The sacro-iliac joint has one other characteristic in which it is different from the intervertebral joints and which is important from a clinical point of view. This is the absence of palpable muscle crossing and controlling the joint, so that there is no muscle in which abnormal tension is diagnostic.

Increased muscle tension in the erector spinae over the upper two sacral segments is commonly found however. Diagnosis, therefore, depends primarily on the finding of loss of movement. The finding of abnormal tension in the lower part of the erector spinae will help when present, so also will tenderness over the posterior sacro-iliac ligament. The clinical finding that symptoms are still present after adequate treatment of the lumbar joints may alert the examiner to a previously unobserved sacro-iliac joint dysfunction. Methods of detection of loss of sacro-iliac movement and for determining the position of the joint will be described in the chapter on examination.

With respect to the finding of tenderness, it is important to distinguish true sacro-iliac tenderness from the tender area very commonly found on the lateral aspect of the posterior spines of the ilium. The latter is caused by a chronic contraction in the origin of the glutei, apparently produced by faulty innervation and may result from spinal joint trouble anywhere in the lumbar region. The specific tender spot in sacro-iliac strains is in the sulcus medial to the inferior part of the posterior superior iliac spine. Tenderness medial to the superior part is more commonly associated with the lumbo-sacral strain.

Before leaving the sacro-iliac joint, mention should be made of Baer's sacro-iliac point which was described many years ago. It is a tender point occurring in the right iliac fossa over the front of the sacro-iliac joint and only a short distance medial to McBurney's appendix point. This point is described as being tender when infection involves the right sacro-iliac joint but may also be found in acute strains of that joint.

Spinal Balance

The concept that the spinal column should be regarded as a single functional unit is at variance with clinical teaching, in spite of the fact that there appears to have been no attempt from within the profession to develop or to learn a method of examining the individual spinal joint as a separate entity. It has already been shown that a sacro-iliac fixation resulting in pelvic torsion can, and does, cause a disturbance of function in the low lumbar region. Experience shows that if a joint becomes stiffened at one end of its travel in the lumbar region, a disturbance of function tends to occur at other levels above and below. This also applies to stiffness occurring primarily either in the thoracic or in the cervical spine. If, for instance, the 2nd lumbar vertebra is forced into the extreme of side bending and rotation to the right, so that the joint between the 2nd and 3rd lumbar vertebrae becomes stiffened in this position, the natural tendency of the spine to adopt a corrective posture will result in the opposite deformity at one or more joints either above or below the lesion.

Again drawing on clinical experience, one finds that unless the primary lesion is relieved, the joints which are secondarily affected will in time tend to stiffen and in many cases will start producing symptoms. These secondary symptom-producing joints are most commonly found in the lower thoracic region, at the cervico-thoracic junction, in the upper cervical spine, or at the joint above or below the original lesion. When the secondary joints do become stiff, they tend themselves to be the cause of a third generation of disturbance of joint function usually at a greater distance from the original lesion.

These considerations suggest that a difference in leg length can be a predisposing cause to persistent trouble from stiffened joints even in the cervical region.

In his training the author was taught to regard as seriously neurotic any patient who complained of pain which started in the low back and ran up the back and down the arm. The basis of this teaching was that no single cause could produce this symptom complex. Considerations of the functional interdependence of the parts of the spine suggest that the symptom complex can have a real organic basis in multiple spinal joint dysfunction. In such a patient muscle spasm, produced at one level by a further strain, could well cause a sufficient upset of the joints at other levels for symptoms to arise from these also.

The Physiological Movements of the Spinal Column

Kapandji[11] describes the automatic rotation of the vertebral column during lateral flexion but does not mention the differences which depend on the degree of flexion or extension of that segment of the spine.

The original observation appears to have been made by Lovett[12] when working on the problem of scoliosis. He found that a column of vertebral bodies separated from its posterior elements behaved as in Kapandji's description. If the column is sidebent, the bodies rotate to the convexity of the sidebend.

When he examined the column of posterior elements however, the rotation was always to the concavity of the sidebend.

Lovett described that, with the intact spine in the living model or the cadaver, the rotation varied. With the spine in extension the rotation was towards the concavity of the sidebend. With the spine flexed the rotation was to the convexity.

Lovett also showed that in extension the facets were held in close apposition but this was not the case in flexion. He concluded that in extension the facets exert a controlling influence because of their close apposition to each other.

Fryette[13] showed that while Lovett's observations were correct, he had omitted to test the movements in the hyperflexed position. Near the limit of flexion the pattern changes once again. The facets assume control and rotation once again is in the direction of the concavity of the sidebend.

These findings were formulated by Fryette into the two laws of spinal motion and this concept has found wide acceptance in the osteopathic profession. For completeness a third law was added.

Law I   With the spine in easy flexion (neutral) the facets are idling and rotation is always to the convexity of the sidebend.

Law II   In extension and in nearly full flexion the facets are in control and rotation must be to the concavity of the sidebend.

Law III   If movement is introduced into a spinal segment in any plane, the range of movement in the other two planes will be reduced.

The clinical significance of this is that if one sidebends the spine in the almost fully flexed position, the rotation will be to the same side (the concavity of the sidebend). If from that point one returns to the erect position suddenly it is possible for the rotation to become jammed rather than untwisting in the normal physiological manner. This may well be one of the mechanisms by which acute back pain is produced.

When the joint becomes jammed with rotation into the concavity of the curve, i.e. in accordance with the 2nd law of spinal motion, it is known as a Type II lesion. Such lesions are commonly traumatic, usually quite acute, and should be treated first. The causative trauma will have occurred either in extension or in hyperflexion of the spine.

When the joint becomes held in a position where rotation is to the convexity of the curve—in accordance with Law I—it is known as a Type I lesion. It is often compensatory and may resolve when the primary joint is treated. Such lesions are often multiple while Type II lesions are nearly always solitary.

In using the terms "jammed" or "held", the author does not wish to beg the question as to which comes first, the stiffness of the joint or the tightness of the muscle.

The Intervertebral Joints
The spinal joint stiffening referred to above is demonstrable both by palpation and by special radiographic techniques. The anatomical and pathological basis for this stiffening is not known. Careful examination of x-rays proves conclusively that in the ordinary sense of the word, there is no displacement. Recent workers have suggested that the explanation may be connected with the intra-articular structures which exist in the facet joints throughout the spine. The existence of these structures has been known for many years but there has been some argument as to their nature and importance.

Schmincke and Santo[14] in 1932 gave a clear description of structures in the cervical region which they considered to be true intra-articular "discs".

Santo[15] later described two different types of structure in the thoracic and lumbar regions, one thin and vascular, the other fibrous with some cartilage cells. He regarded the former as a synovial fold and the latter as an articular "disc".

Töndury[16] described similar structures and regarded them as derived from the synovial membrane but he also found a connection between some of the structures and the extra-articular pad of fat.

Zaccheo and Reale[17] investigated 20 vertebral columns from infancy to old age and described 3 distinct types of intra-articular structures, including not only those reported by Schmincke, Santo and Töndury but also what they consider to be a true meniscus. The other structures they described as synovial folds and fatty bodies respectively.

They regard the meniscus as having the typical functions of shock absorbtion and padding to produce conformity of shape on movement. The other structures are thought to be concerned with production of synovial fluid and with the filling up of spaces left above and below the joint on flexion movement.

It seems conceivable that injury to these structures, small as they are, could result in an upset of joint function and be responsible for symptoms.

Dörr[18] also studied the anatomy of the intervertebral joint in detail and described similar structures as well as interlaminar bursae found in the cervical region. He discusses the function of the various structures and concludes "We were unable to discover from our studies whether 'trapped discs' are the cause of backache" (author's translation) but goes on to compare them with the menisci in the knee joint and deduces that if a meniscus is first trapped by positioning and then moved, it could cause pain by traction on the capsule.

Lewin et al.[19] review the literature and describe further investigations into the anatomy of the intervertebral joint. They point out that the meniscus-like structures are in fact true menisci because they are found at all ages including the new-born. They point to the lack of synovial cells over the majority of the surface of the menisci as an indication that these structures actually bear weight.

Lewin and his co-workers also investigated the movements and point out that the intervertebral joint must be regarded as a triad consisting of the disc and the two apophyseal joints. On flexion and extension the facets slide in the sagittal plane while the nucleus displaces dorsally or ventrally, on side bending the facets slide in opposite directions and the nucleus displaces away from the direction of flexion. "If any rotation occurs in the lumbar spine, it happens in spite of the fact that the lumbar joints are designed to prevent rotation . . . an attempt to impose a rotatory movement on the lumbar spine subjects the lumbar vertebral joints to their greatest loading and at the same time exerts a shearing movement on the intervertebral disc."

It is an observed fact that treatments directed to obtaining relaxation of the abnormally tight muscle can in some circumstances be highly successful. This success suggests that one of the main factors in producing and maintaining the loss of motion in the joint is the abnormal tension in the muscle.

The Disc

The annulus is composed of rings of fibrocartilage, eighteen to twenty in number in an adult, set at an angle to each other. Posteriorly the lamellae run vertically and are parallel bands, but at their lateral extremities they are interlaced with the oblique fibres. In infants the lamellae are less distinct and fewer in number, but become more clearly differentiated and increase in numbers until about the end of the growth period. Increase in thickness of the annulus is partly at the expense of the nucleus and partly by appositional growth from the long ligaments.[20] The ends of the fibres forming the lamellae are firmly attached to the bone and in front are reinforced by the strong anterior common ligament. Both above and below the disc, these fibres tend to curl inwards around the nucleus before being attached to the bone. The unaltered nucleus is not a pulp, but a translucent gel containing a three-dimensional network of fine collagen fibrils.[21]

Hirsch[22] found that the nucleus "is not a watery gel but is composed of highly organised material." He also described numerous collagen fibres in the nuclei of children and young persons surrounded by chondromucoid elements. Hirsch and Schajowicz[20] found radiating ruptures in many autopsy discs. When complete they contained highly vascular connective tissue which had grown out from the long ligament. Concentric cracks or cavities were even more common but were thought to be physiological.

In normal discograms Lindblom[23] showed that the disc contained cavities which could be filled with contrast medium. These cavities were principally above and below the nucleus, between it and the vertebral end plates. In the abnormal the cavity was more extensive, extending backwards close to the vertebra. This was apparently caused by tearing of the fibres attaching the annulus to bone and resulted from loss of elasticity of the posterior annulus secondary to the radiating cracks which appear in degenerating discs.

The avascularity of the disc has been commented on by many workers and appears to be complete except for the most superficial part of the annulus.[2] No nerve fibres have been demonstrated in the disc other than by Roofe[24] who found them in the posterior part of the annulus. These appear to arise from the sinu-vertebral nerve of Lushka.

The Atlanto-Occipital and Atlanto-Axial Joints

The structure and function of the intervertebral joints from the lumbosacral up to that between the 2nd and 3rd cervical are essentially similar throughout although there are marked individual variations in the range of mobility. In the thoracic region there is the added complication of the neighbouring costo-vertebral articulations with their associated muscles and ligaments. Between the skull and the 1st cervical and between the 1st and 2nd cervical vertebrae there is a profound change in structure which is necessitated by the change in function at this level. The atlanto-occipital joint is designed to give a maximum of flexion and extension movement in the sagittal plane with some sidebending. Werne[25] investigated the movement of the atlanto-occipital and atlanto-axial joints and concluded that rotatory movement did not occur at the atlanto-occipital nor did tilting to the side occur at the atlanto-axial joint. He said that the two joints should be regarded as a functional unit permitting flexion and extension in the upper and, to a less extent, at the lower joint and permitting sidebending at the upper joint and rotation at the lower joint. He did, however, conclude that "tilting and turning are always combined" even if they occur at separate anatomical sites. Fielding[26] points out that vertical approximation is also possible at the atlanto-axial joint.

In neither joint is there an intervertebral disc, nor is there any other structure that can cause actual pressure on nerve or nerve root in a confined space as can happen in the typical intervertebral joint with a postero-lateral disc protrusion.

Similarly, in the sacro-iliac joint there can be no question of nerve pressure from a disc protrusion. The symptoms and signs which can only be produced by actual nerve compression therefore do not occur in lesions of these three joints. Stiffness, local pain and referred pain and tenderness can and do occur however, and are comparable in every respect to the similar symptoms arising in typical intervertebral joints.

Examples of case records in which the clinical evidence pointed strongly to lesions of the atlanto-occipital and sacro-iliac joints as the cause of referred symptoms are given in the Appendix (Cases 1–9).

The Innervation of the Intervertebral Joints

The innervation of the structures of and around the interverte-bral joints was investigated by Pedersen et al.[27] and more recently by Wyke[45]. Their findings are basically similar. Wyke described:

1 Branches of the posterior primary rami supplying the apophyseal joints, the periosteum and the related fasciae of the surfaces of the vertebral bodies and their arches, the interspinous ligaments and the blood vessels;
2 Pain afferents in the sinu-vertebral nerves having endings in the posterior longitudinal and flaval ligaments, the dura mater and the surrounding fatty tissue, the epidural veins and the periosteum of the spinal canal;
3 A plexus of nerve fibres which surrounds the paravertebral venous system. Receptors supplied by these nerve fibres are found throughout almost the same area as those supplied by the sinu-vertebral nerve. All the pain afferent fibres are small, either thinly or not at all myelinated.

The Muscles of the Shoulder Girdle and Upper Trunk

The muscles of the upper back are arranged in three groups.[28] The superficial group arc the muscles connecting the shoulder girdle to the trunk and consist of the trapezius, latissimus dorsi, levator scapulae, and the rhomboids. These have all migrated caudalwards and their innervation is derived from cervical segments. Tender areas in these muscles can, therefore, be expected to be associated with disturbances of cervical nerve function. The intermediate group consists of the serratus posterior superior (and inferior). These arc muscles of respiration which have migrated backwards. They are innervated by the ventral rami of the thoracic nerves and deep to these are the muscles of the spinal column itself which are innervated by the dorsal rami. Any disturbance in the intermediate or deep muscles can therefore be expected to be associated with an alteration in function of the thoracic, rather than cervical nerves.

The clinical importance of this is that muscle tenderness between the midline and the vertebral border of the scapula up to the back of the 1st rib can, if superficial, be due to a cervical joint disturbance or, if deep, to trouble in the thoracic spine. The distinction of the depth at which the muscle is tender may be impossible to make and therefore the examination must include both cervical and thoracic regions.

Range of Mobility of Individual Spinal Joints

Cervical
Measurement of the range of flexion-extension movement in the individual cervical joints has been undertaken by a number of authors. Penning[29] gives the figures quoted by several authors including himself, describes his technique and discusses the results. The technique he used was to take lateral radiographs in the fully flexed and fully extended positions of the neck and a third view with the head fully flexed on the neck, but the neck itself only partly flexed. This was necessary because he found that full flexion of the neck tended to cause a deflexion at the atlanto-occipital joint in order to get the chin out of the way. The measurement of the angle of movement was done by superimposing each vertebra in turn and marking the film in a similar way to that described by Troup[30] for the lumbar spine (page 33).

Penning's average results are very similar to those of other recent workers but the range of individual variation is great in all the series published. The results obtained by Penning himself are set out in Table I.

Table I Range of Sagittal Motion in the Cervical Spine (Penning)

Joint	Range in Degrees	Average
C0–1	6 to 30	—
C1–2	3 to 35	—
C2–3	5 to 16	$12\frac{1}{2}$
C3–4	13 to 26	18
C4–5	15 to 29	20
C5–6	16 to 29	$21\frac{1}{2}$
C6–7	6 to 25	$15\frac{1}{2}$
C7–T1	4 to 12	8

Thoracic

Motion is restricted in the thoracic region in all directions when compared to either of the other regions. There appear to have been no experimental studies of the range of movement of the individual joints. There is a relatively abrupt change in mobility between the C6–7 and the T1–2 joints, but a major part of this change occurs between the C6–7 and C7–T1 joints. Penning's average movement for the latter being only half of the average of the former.

The transition at the thoraco-lumbar junction takes place at a joint which differs structurally from either the thoracic joint above or the lumbar joint below. The structural difference lies in the shape of the articular processes which, at this level, have been likened by Davis[31] to a carpenter's mortice. This joint is most commonly found between the 11th and 12th thoracic but can be either at that between T10 and 11 or, rather more commonly, at that between T12 and L1. Owing to the shape of the articular processes at this level movements other than flexion-extension are much restricted and flexion-extension is also less free than at any of the joints below.

Lumbar

A very full discussion of the literature and fresh experimental work is reported by Troup[30]. He examined statistically a variety of different methods of measuring the movement between individual lumbar vertebrae as shown by x-rays in the flexed and in the extended position.

By statistical analysis Troup was able to show that a method of marking angles by successive superimposition of the outlines of the individual lumbar vertebrae was very significantly superior to any of the methods which involve the drawing of lines on the films to mark the inclination of the individual vertebrae. The method of superimposition of x-rays was originally described by Begg and Falconer[32] and was that used by Penning in the cervical spine.

Most other workers who have recorded the range of movement of the lumbar spine by radiological methods have relied on the measurement of angles between lines drawn on the x-rays designed to show the inclination of the individual vertebra. The inaccuracy appears to be due in part to the difficulty in determining the exact position of the points between which the line should be drawn and in part to the fact that a double error is involved as for each measurement two lines have to be drawn.

In Troup's modification of Begg and Falconer's superimposition method, the outlines of the sacrum on the two x-rays are first superimposed. The x-rays are, of course, taken in the lateral projection, one with the spine flexed and the other with it extended. Care must be taken to see that the relationship of the tube head, pelvis and cassette are standardised.

With the two sacra superimposed a line is drawn on the underneath film marking one of the edges of the upper film. The upper film is then realigned so that the outlines of the 5th lumbar vertebrae are superimposed. A second line is then drawn marking the same edge of the upper film on the film underneath and the process is repeated for each of the lumbar vertebrae. Finally, the angles between the successive lines are measured with a protractor.

Troup[30] points out that the exposure to radiation involved in taking films of the lumbar spine is sufficient to be a hazard, the more so because of the proximity of the sex glands. He therefore regarded the method as unjustified in the normal and the figures which he gives are based on radiographic examination of patients with lumbar symptoms for whom x-ray examination was needed on clinical grounds. It is likely, therefore, that his figures are somewhat lower than would be obtained by a similar examination of strictly normal spines.

The means and standard deviations of the estimated movements at the individual joints in Troup's series are set out in Table II.

A somewhat surprising result shown in Troup's figures is that in the upper two lumbar joints there is a tendency for a

Table II Range of Sagittal Motion in the Lumbar Spine (Troup)

Joint	Full flexion to full extension		Full flexion to erect position	
	Mean	*SD*	*Mean*	*SD*
L1–2	7.5	2.3	8.6	1.7
L2–3	10.5	3.4	10.3	3.6
L3–4	11.1	2.8	11.2	2.5
L4–5	12.9	4.0	12.0	3.9
L5–S1	11.0	3.9	9.0	6.4

flexor movement to occur between the erect and the fully extended posture of the body. In some subjects there was a flexor movement in the upper two lumbar joints when the spine was extended beyond the erect position. This can be compared to the deflexion of the atlanto-occipital joint mentioned above.

Also in 1968, Froning and Frohman[33] investigated the range of movement at the individual lumbar joints in patients and in people supposedly normal. The figures for the normal are reproduced in Table III and it will be seen that figures for the L4–5 and L5–S1 joints are significantly greater than those given by Troup.

Troup's observations were on those with lumbar symptoms and it is well known that such symptoms more commonly arise from the lower two lumbar joints than from the upper three. It is, therefore, to be expected that Troup's figures for patients with symptoms would be lower particularly with respect to the L4–5 and L5–S1 joints than those obtained from supposedly normal people. The requirements for normality as laid down by Froning and Frohman were a balanced standing posture, negative neurological findings, absence of sciatic nerve tenderness or pain on stretching the nerve and no x-ray changes either in the osseous structures or in the disc spaces. They point out that the numbers in the various age groups are small owing to the difficulty in obtaining a sufficient number who fulfilled these strict conditions. A striking conclusion to be drawn from these figures is that among those who fulfil these criteria for normality, the loss of motion with increasing age is remarkably slight.

In their study of abnormal lumbar spines Froning and Frohman found that an increase of motion was common in levels adjacent to those showing restriction. A similar observation was recorded by Jirout[34]. This appears to be the explanation of the

Table III Range of Sagittal Motion in the Lumbar Spine (Froning and Frohman)

Number of Cases	Ages	L5	L4	L3	L2	L1
5	20–29	18	17	14	14	13
11	30–39	17	16	14	10	9
8	40–49	16	16	13	10	8
5	50–59	16	15	12	11	7
1	60–70	16	14	10	10	6
	Average	17	16	13	11	9

finding of individual joint stiffness in a segment of the spine with normal overall mobility.

Froning and Frohman also found that after partial disc removal a statistically significant proportion of cases with good results showed restriction of motion but those with bad results retained greater mobility. The reasons for this were not discovered.

For a full discussion on the physiology of the joints of the spine see Kapandji but note that he appeared to be unaware either of Penning's observations on movements of the atlanto-occipital joints or of Froning and Frohman's observation on lumbar movements in the normal ageing spine.

The Autonomic Nervous System

The precise role of both sympathetic and parasympathetic nerves in the appreciation of pain remains to be worked out. Experience with many clinical cases indicates that pain reference often occurs from certain spinal segments to parts of the body with which that segment appears to have no nerve connection other than in the autonomic system. Bingham[35] thought that there was evidence to suggest that pain actually travelled in sympathetic afferent fibres. The problem is discussed by Barnes[36] who concludes that it is unlikely on the grounds that:

1 No sensory change of any kind has ever been demonstrated in a sympathectomised limb;
2 In spinal lesions where the cord is damaged below the lowest sympathetic outflow, the sympathetic innervation of the lower limb is intact but there is a total insensibility of the area supplied by somatic nerves arising in the segments below the damage;
3 (with special reference to the pain of causalgia) That a low

spinal anaesthetic will relieve this pain before there is any effect on the sympathetic fibres.

On clinical grounds alone there is ample evidence to show that some disturbance of sympathetic function can be associated with the production of referred pain in certain sites. Therefore, the level of origin of sympathetic fibres to the various parts of the upper and lower limbs is of interest to the surgeon who is called upon to find the source of certain types of referred pain. The level of the sympathetic outflow supplying the head, neck and trunk is generally better known but that to the head and neck is included because it seems likely that abnormal sympathetic activity is one of the major factors in the production of some headaches and, if these are the result of a spinal joint abnormality, it is important to know at which level to look.

Table IV Sympathetic Innervation of More Important Structures (based on Mitchell[37])

Structure	Location of pre-ganglionic cells	Chief efferent pathways
Eyes	T1–2	Internal carotid plexus to ciliary nerves or along vessels
Vessels of head	T1–2(and 3)	Vascular plexuses
Upper limbs	T2(3) to T6(7)	Rami communicates to roots of brachial plexus
Heart	T1–4(5)	Cardiac sympathetic nerves to cardiac plexus
Stomach	T6–9(10)	Via coeliac plexus
Kidneys	T12(11) to L1(2)	Via coeliac plexus
Bladder and uterus	T12(11) to L1(2)	Lumbar splanchnic nerves
Lower limbs	T11(10) to L2	Rami communicantes to lumbar and sacral nerves

Mitchell[37] states that the afferent pain fibres from the cervix uteri, base of bladder, prostate and rectum are carried in the pelvic splanchnic nerves and their cells are located in the dorsal root ganglia of the 2nd, 3rd and 4th sacral nerves.

Neuwirth[38] reviews relatively recent work on the anatomy of the sympathetic nervous system in the neck, most of which was done in France by Laruelle[39], Delmas *et al.*[40], and Tinel[41]. Laruelle describes that he demonstrated sympathetic cell bodies in the mediolateral grey matter at the base of the anterior horns at the levels of the spinal cord segments of C4, 5, 6, 7 and 8. The preganglionic fibres from these are said to proceed with the somatic motor fibres in the ventral roots from C5 to T1 inclusive, and some are said to synapse in the small ganglia found on the sympathetic plexus around the vertebral artery. Others traverse these ganglia, join the plexus and by this means, reach the cerivco-thoracic group. According to Tinel the fibres of C5 join the carotid plexus and are distributed to the subclavian plexus and thereby reach the arm and the nerves of the brachial plexus. Those from C7 go to the cardioaortic plexus, to the thoracic branches of the axillary and subclavian arteries and the phrenic nerves.

By these findings Neuwirth sought to explain:

1 The relief of headaches and facial pain which can follow treatment of the neck;
2 Similar results with what he terms dysaesthesias and vascular pain in the upper extremity, and
3 Pain in the upper part of the back and anterior chest wall simulating angina.

Unfortunately, this work which was done in France has not yet been confirmed by other workers. The volume of the sympathetic outflow at these levels appears to be small and it seems likely that the true explanation involves some other nervous mechanism.

Sensory Distribution of the Spinal Nerve Roots

It has been known for many years that the distribution of sensory fibres to the skin from the various spinal nerve roots does not correspond to the distribution of any of the individual cutaneous nerves, except over the trunk where the correspondence is fair. Head[42] studied the distribution of the cutaneous hyperalgesia and the vesicles in cases of Herpes Zoster. As the result of this study he was able to draw a map showing the distribution of the various spinal nerves with respect to the skin of the body. At about the same time Sherrington[43] mapped the distribution of nerve fibres by a different technique.

Sherrington worked on the Rhesus monkey which, at least for the head, neck, upper limbs and trunk, has a very similar

nerve distribution to that of man. In his experiments the posterior roots of a number of nerves were cut on either side of the
one under investigation. The sensation remaining was then
mapped by a painful stimulus applied to the area, note being
made of a minimal motor response. The chief difference between
the results obtained by Sherrington and those obtained by Head
lay in the fact that Sherrington's areas were considerably larger
and indicated major overlap. Head's were discreet, with almost
no overlap.

The configuration of the lumbar spine is different in the Rhesus
monkey and the human, and there appears to be some difference
in the distribution of the lumbar and sacral nerves to the lower
limbs so that the correspondence of the areas in the lower limb
is less good. Both Head and Sherrington found that the areas
which were mapped in the more distal parts of the limb were
separated from the spine by skin which apparently had no
sensory innervation from the spinal segment under investigation.
This led to the belief that the growing limb bud drew away from
the trunk all the sensory supply of the nerves at these levels (the
loop theory). Much more recently Keegan and Garrett[44] have
reinvestigated the problem by a method more similar to Head's
than to that of Sherrington. The results published by other
investigators have not been essentially different from those of
Head or Sherrington.

Keegan and Garrett showed that in cases of disc protrusion
it is very unusual for more than one nerve root to be affected
and that in cases with compression of one nerve root an area of
hypoalgesia can be marked out in a repeatable fashion, even
when conduction in the sensory fibres has not been completely
abolished. Their technique briefly, was to use a pin scratch of
firmness adjusted to cause no more than a mildly unpleasant
sensation in the hypoalgesic area. Using this method they
found " . . . that the dermatomes continue unbroken from dorsal
midline to their termination in the limb, and that they have
developed in a very different manner than postulated in the
loop theory."

The charts which they drew are reproduced in Fig. 2.

During the course of the investigation Keegan and Garrett
found that they were able to map out, not only the main
distribution of the individual nerve root, but also a fainter
overlap distribution extending often an inch of two on either
side of the main distribution. It seems reasonable to think that
the larger overlap distribution corresponds to Sherrington's area

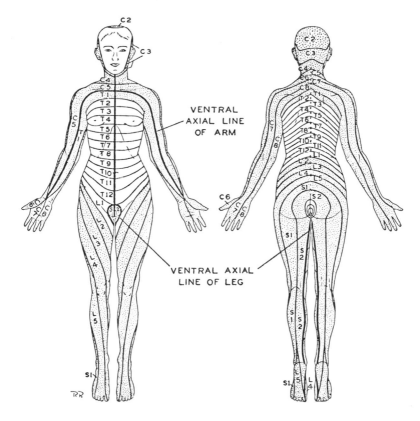

Fig. 2 Dermatome chart of the human body drawn by Keegan and Garrett.

and the smaller to those outlined by Head. A comparison of the areas with those mapped by Head (Fig. 3) will show that in the distal part of the limb there is a very fair correspondence between the two. Fortunately, from the clinician's point of view, the proximal areas of the various dermatomes are of much less importance than the distal ones, about which there is fair general agreement.

When considering possible causes of pain in the buttock it is important to remember that the skin of the buttock is in part innervated by the cutaneous branches of the posterior primary division of the 11th and 12th thoracic nerves. This may be one mechanism by which pain in the buttock can be produced by problems in the low thoracic spine.

40

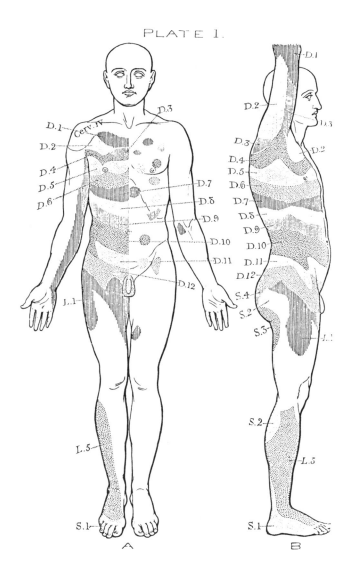

Fig. 3 Dermatome chart drawn by Head showing both the total area and the maxima.

PLATE II.

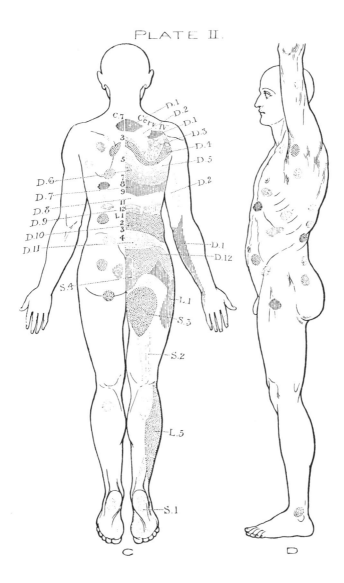

C

D

REFERENCES

1 Mixter, W. J. and Barr, J. S. (1934), Rupture of the intervertebral disc, *New Eng. J. Med.* **211**, 210–215.
2 Armstrong, J. R. (1965), *Lumbar Disc Lesions*, 3rd Ed., London, Livingstone.
3 Brooke, R. (1924), The sacro-iliac joint, *J. Anat.* **58**, 299–305.
4 Pitkin, H. C. and Pheasant, H. C. (1936), Sacrarthrogenic telalgia, *J. Bone Jt. Surg.* **18**, 111–133, 365–374.
5 Gray, H. (1938), Sacro-iliac joint pain, *Int. Cl.* **2**, 54–96.
6 *Cunningham's Textbook of Anatomy* (1964), 10th Ed., London, Oxford University Press.
7 Weisl, H. (1955), Movement of the sacro-iliac joint, *Acta anat.* **23**, 80–91.
8 *Gray's Anatomy, Descriptive and Applied* (1958), 32nd Ed., London, Longmans.
9 Kapandji, I. A., The physiology of the joints, **3**, 70, Churchill Livingstone.
10 Schunke, G. B. (1938), Anatomy and development of the sacro-iliac joint in men, *Anat. Rec.* **72**, 313–331.
11 Kapandji, I. A., ibid. p. 42.
12 Lovett, Robert W., M.D. (1) The mechanics of lateral curvature of the spine, *Boston MSJ*, 1900 XCLII, 622–627. (2) The study of the mechanics of the spine, *Am. J. Anat.* II, 1902–1903, 457–462.
13 Fryette, H. H., *The Principles of Osteopathic Technique*, 1954, Academy of Applied Osteopathy.
14 Schmincke, A. and Santo, E. (1932), Zur normalen und pathologischen Anatomie der Halswirbelsäule, *Zbl. Path.* **55**, 369–372.
15 Santo, E. (1935), Zur Entwicklungsgeschichte und Histologie der Zwischenscheiben in den kleinen Gelenken. *Zeitschr. f. Anat. u. Entwicklungsgesch.* **104**, 623–634.
16 Töndury, G. (1940), Beitrag zur Kenntnis der kleinen Wirbelgelenke. *Zeitschr. f. Anat. u. Entwicklungsgesch.* **110**. 568–575.
17 Zaccheo, D. and Reale, E. (1955), Contributo alla cognoscenza delle articolazioni tra i processi articolari delle vertebre dell'uomo. *Archivio di Anatomia* **61**, 1–16.
18 Dörr, W. M. (1958), Über die Anatomie der Wirbelgelenke. *Arch. F. orthop. u. Unfall-Chir.* **50**, 222–234.
19 Lewin, T., Moffett, B. and Viidik, A. (1961), The morphology of the Lumbar Synovial Intervertebral joints. *Acta Morphologica Neerlando-Scandinavia.* **4**, 299–319.
20 Hirsch, C. and Schajowicz, F. (1952), Studies on structural change in the lumbar annulus fibrosus, *Acta orthopaed. scand.* **22**, 184–231.
21 Sylven, B. (1951), On the biology of the nucleus pulposus, *Acta orthopaed. scand.* **20**, 275–279.
22 Hirsch, C. (1959), Studies on the pathology of back pain, *J. Bone Jt. Surg.* **41B**, 237–247.
23 Lindblom, K. (1951), Technique and results of disc puncture, *Acta orthopaed. scand.* **20**, 315–326.
24 Roofe, P. G. (1939), Innervation of annulus fibrosus, *Arch. Path.* **27**, 201–211.
25 Werne, S. (1959), The cranio vertebral joints, *Acta orthopaed. scand.* **28**, 165–173.
26 Fielding, J. W. (1957), Cineroentgenography of the normal cervical spine,

J. Bone Jt. Surg. **39A**, 1280–1288.
27 Pedersen, H. E., Blunck, G. F. J. and Gardner, E. (1956), Anatomy of lumbo-sacral posterior rami, *J. Bone Jt. Surg.* **38A**, 377–391.
28 *Grant's Method of Anatomy* (1965), 7th Ed., Baltimore, Williams and Wilkins.
29 Penning, L. (1968), *Functional Pathology of the Cervical Spine*, Excerpta Medica Foundation, Amsterdam.
30 Troup, J. D. G. (1968), Ph.D. Thesis, London University.
31 Davis, P. R. (1955), The thoraco-lumbar mortice joint, *J. Anat.* **89**, 370–371.
32 Begg, C. and Falconer, M. A. (1949), Plain radiography in intraspinal protrusions of intervertebral discs, *J. Bone Jt. Surg.* **36**, 225.
33 Froning, E. C. and Frohman, B. (1968), Motion of the lumbo-sacral spine after laminectomy and spine fusion, *J. Bone Jt. Surg.* **50A**, 897–918.
34 Jirout, J. (1955), Studies in the dynamics of the spine, *Excerpta Acta Radiol.* **46**, Fasc.
35 Bingham, J. A. W. (1948), Some problems of causalgic pain, *Brit. Med. J.* **2**, 334–338.
36 Barnes, R. (1954), Causalgia in Peripheral Nerve Injuries, M.R.C. Special Reports Series 282, London, H.M.S.O.
37 Mitchell, G. (1953), *The Anatomy of the Autonomic Nervous System*, Edinburgh, Livingstone.
38 Neuwirth, E. (1960), Current concepts of the cervical portion of the sympathetic nervous system, *J. Lancet* **80**, 337–338.
39 Laruelle, M. L. (1940), Les bases anatomiques du système autonomic cortical et bulbo-spinal, *Rev. Neurol.* **72**, 349–360.
40 Delmas, J., Laux, G. and Guerrier, Y. (1947), Comment atteindre les fibres préganglionaires du membre superieur, *Gaz. méd. Fr.* **59**, 703.
41 Tinel, J. (1937), *La System Nerveux Vegetatif*, Paris, Masseon.
42 Head, H. (1893), Disturbances of sensation with special reference to the pain of visceral disease, *Brain* **16**, 1–133, 339–480.
43 Sherrington, C. S. (1893), Experiments in examination of the peripheral distribution of the fibres of the posterior roots of some spinal nerves, *Phil. Trans.* **B184**, 641–763; **B190**, 45–187.
44 Keegan, J. J., and Garrett, F. D. (1948), Segmental sensory nerve distribution, *Anat. Rec.* **102**, 409–437.
45 Wyke, B. (1970), The neurological basis of thoracic spinal pain, *Rheumatology and Physical Medicine* **10**, 356–366.

3

Examination

General Considerations
The Pelvis and Lumbar Spine

In order to simplify description of examination and treatment techniques in this book the patient will be designated by the female gender and the examiner by the male.

The Spinal Joint Lesion

Before one learns a new technique of examination, it is important to know for what one is looking. This is further discussed in a later chapter. For present purposes the characteristic signs of a spinal joint lesion for which manipulative treatment is appropriate are that the joint shows restricted movement and that the muscles over one side of the joint show excess tension.

Spinal joints when damaged have the property of losing part or all of their mobility. This, of course, also tends to happen to the more easily accessible joints, the more so if they are neglected after injury. As in the case of peripheral joints that have become stiff after injury, spinal joints with reduced mobility can remain symptomless for long periods, even up to many years. The precise reason why they should suddenly start to give trouble after remaining symptomless for such periods is a matter that could well be the subject of future research. Experience strongly suggests that, with one exception, stiffened joints over which there is no detectable excess tension in the muscles are unlikely to be the source of major symptoms. The exception is the sacro-iliac joint which is not closely bridged by its controlling muscles and any excess tension in them is not so easily felt by the examining finger.

It may not be possible to restore to a damaged joint a full range of movement. For the relief of symptoms, however, it is usually enough to restore some movement and to obtain release of the abnormal tension in the associated muscles. At this point it is perhaps appropriate to emphasize once again that there is no "little bone out of place" and that the manipulation is not in any way designed to put back into place any dislocated or subluxated bone. The joint is held in such a way that movement in at least one direction is demonstrably restricted. Movement in other directions may be normal. This accounts for the relative normality of the x-rays.

The objective signs of stiffness and excess tension in the muscles are of much greater importance than the subjective sign of tenderness. It is usual for the examiner to be able to assess the response of any given patient quite quickly and to estimate the value in any particular case of the subjective signs. In those in whom these signs can be expected to be valuable, the presence of tenderness at the same site as the excess muscle tension is a useful confirmatory sign of the presence of a joint lesion for which treatment is likely to be helpful.

The accurate appreciation of joint stiffness and, even more, that of excess tension in the muscles requires training and in some people, even with constant practice, this training takes a long time. The necessity for this training is not always appreciated and its neglect has often led to the impression among non-manipulators that the manipulator is imagining the abnormality and that he spends his time treating something that does not exist. The difficulty can perhaps be compared to that of a novice trying to read Braille. Distinguishing the pattern of the raised dots is easy for those who have had sufficient practice. It is quite impossible for those like myself who have not, and, to the beginner, the idea that it might be possible seems almost unbelievable. It is a good thing that there are many patients in whom the stiffness and the muscle spasm can be felt easily enough to convice all except the most bigoted disbelievers.

The Barrier

A normal joint will move through a certain range of active motion. Beyond the end of what the muscles can do actively, there is a small additional passive range. From that point on there has to be damage to bone or ligament and a subluxation or dislocation occurs. This can be illustrated by the diagrams in Fig. 4. The end of the active range is known as the physiological barrier (B, B_1) and the end of the passive as the anatomical barrier (A, A_1).

So far we have been discussing normal joints. In the abnormal there is restriction of movement in one or more directions and a

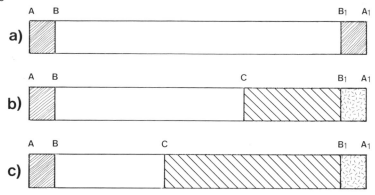

Fig. 4 The barrier concept. (a) Represents a normal joint. The range of physiological movement is represented as the distance between B and B_1. The total possible movement is that between A and A_1. The ranges A, B and A_1, B_1 are the passive ranges at either end. (b) Represents a joint with restricted motion. The available movement is now only from B to C with the passive range A, B. (c) Represents a major restriction, the remaining range being only about $\frac{1}{3}$ of normal. (Kimberly [1])

new barrier is formed (C). The restriction may be major so that only a small range of movement remains, or it may be minor so that the range is only a little less than normal.

The reasons for the existence of a pathological barrier will be discussed later. The barrier is of great clinical importance because it is an objective sign which can be detected, treated and found to be removed. There are several methods of removing the barrier and two main ones will be described. The significance of the success of a variety of different treatments will also be discussed later.

Somatic Dysfunction

As a result of agreement between the government and the Osteopathic profession in the U.S.A. the term somatic dysfunction has been introduced as the proper description of the spinal joint disturbance and its associated complications. This replaces the maligned term "osteopathic lesion" and has been defined as: "Impaired or altered function of related components of the somatic (body framework) system: skeletal, arthrodial, and myofascial structures; and related vascular, lymphatic and neural elements."

General Examination

It is always wise to do a thorough examination of any patient seen for the first time. Patients are sometimes referred for back trouble when they are suffering from hip disease and for hip troubles when they have nothing more difficult than a back lesion that will respond to treatment. Ulnar neuritis can be due to irritation of the nerve at the level of the proximal row of the carpus, to irritation in the groove behind the epicondyle of the humerus, to root irritation by cervical joint lesions or even to a cervical rib. The finding of stiffness in the lower cervical joints does not excuse the practitioner from excluding other possible causes of nerve irritation.

At least a limited neurological examination on the first visit is always a wise precaution. In some patients it should be repeated at least in part in order to assess progress; the more so if there is any question of deterioration.

The Musculo-Skeletal System

Referred pain is very common and often it does not follow in the expected pattern of the dermatome, myotome, or sclerotome. Partly for this reason when dealing with symptoms arising from the musculo-skeletal system the most important thing is to look for loss of function. In some cases it will be found that the loss of function is not at any of the levels which one would expect to be segmentally related to the symptoms.

Because of his own past experience the author recognizes that this concept is one which is alien to the thinking of most orthodox physicians. Unfortunately, most of us have been taught to believe that referred pain is necessarily related segmentally to its site of origin. To anyone who finds this concept unacceptable I would ask that you go along with the idea as a possibility and observe how it develops.

The work of Dr. Janet Travell and Dr. John Mennell[2] on the pain patterns produced by myofascial trigger points does show that the referred pain from these points is not always in segmental relation to the trigger point. Mennell gives a series of diagrams which could with advantage be in the office of every physician practising in this field. He also describes one method of treatment for these pain producing lesions.

In order to save time it is helpful to divide the examination into two parts.

1 An overall screening examination that will show up regions where mobility or muscle tone are abnormal.
2 A detailed examination of the abnormal regions to make a

precise diagnosis as to the particular joint involved, the direction of the restriction of motion in that joint, and the location of any abnormal tension.

The Overall Screening Examination

When examining a patient with pain thought to be of spinal origin, it is wise to begin by observing the function of the lower extremities in walking as well as in standing and lying. In simple walking look for asymmetry in size, range of motion, and muscle tension. When examining for difference in level on the two sides it is useful to use the information from your proprioceptors as well as from your eyes.

In these examinations you should be aware of which is your master eye. When looking for small alterations of position of this nature it is important that the master eye should be over the midline of the patient.

To determine your master eye, make a circle with the index finger and thumb of one hand and hold it out in front at arm's length. With both eyes open observe what is seen clearly through the circle. Then close each eye in turn. When the object originally seen remains in view, you are looking with your master eye. When the object changes the master eye is closed.

Standing Examination

1 Static—First, from behind look for the levels of:
   (a) the gluteal folds
   (b) the trochanters
   (c) the iliac crests
   (d) the shoulders
   (e) the scapulae
   Look also for any tilting of the head.
   Secondly, from the sides:
   (a) are the cervical, thoracic and lumbar curves normal or are they exaggerated or flattened?
   (b) is the head held in front of the gravity line? The vertical from the ear should pass through the shoulder, hip, knee and ankle.
   Thirdly, from the front:
   (a) look for the height of the anterior superior iliac spines.
   (b) look for the shoulder height.
   (c) look for rotation of the face and tilting of the head.
2 With movement—
   The patient must be instructed to keep the knees straight

because failure to do this will materially affect the findings.

(a) Flexion—extension movement

Note the range of forward flexion and of extension and whether these movements are smooth or whether there is a catch.

(b) Standing forward flexion test—This is a test for limitation of movement in the sacro-iliac joints. When the test is positive the movement of the posterior superior iliac spine (PSIS) will begin earlier on that side and will usually be greater. (Fig. 5)

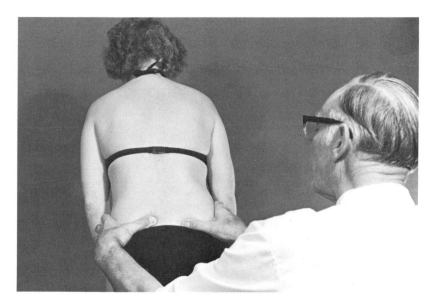

Fig. 5 The standing forward flexion test. Note that the examiner's left thumb has ridden up compared to the right indicating restricted movement of the sacrum on the ilium on the left side.

1 The patient stands with the knees straight and feet level but about six inches apart.
2 You stand or sit behind her.
3 Monitor the movement of the PSIS with your thumbs.
4 The patient bends forwards slowly.
5 Observe which PSIS starts to move first and which moves furthest.

NOTE:

(1) When the sacro-iliac joint does not move properly, flexion of the trunk (and sacrum) will cause the ilium

to move sooner than if the joint were mobile.

(2) The thumbs may either be placed horizontally so that the pad bridges the sulcus between the PSIS and the back of the sacrum or they may be brought up from below to rest beneath the ledge under the posterior superior iliac spine.

(3) Unilateral tightness of the hamstring muscles destroys the value of this test.

(c) Side bending—

Have the patient bend fully first to one side and then to the other with her knees straight. Observe any segments of the spine which do not move normally (this observation can be made up to the mid thoracic spine in this position).

(d) Hip drop test—

Some people find it easier to interpret the information from this more localized side bending. (Fig. 6)

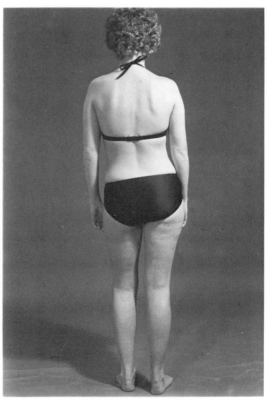

Fig. 6 The hip drop test. Flexion of the left knee allows the left side of the pelvis to drop producing sidebending in the lumbar spine.

1 The patient stands erect as before.
2 You stand or sit behind her.
3 Have her stand on one leg and flex the opposite knee allowing that hip to drop.
4 Repeat on the other side.
5 Observe the smoothness of the lumbar curve to each side, the position of its apex and any difference in the angle or distance dropped by the hips.

Seated Examination

(a) Sitting forward flexion test—
The test for the sacro-iliac movement is repeated with the patient sitting. The information is complementary to the standing flexion test but the results may be different. They are no longer affected by unilateral hamstring tightness and different forces operate because the weight is now being taken on the ischial tuberosities.

The patient sits on a stool with her feet on the floor. If she sits on the side of the examination table she must have a stool to support her feet. Her knees must be far enough apart to allow full flexion of the trunk.

The test is performed in the same manner as the standing test.

If the feet are not supported it is easy for the patient to fall forwards off the table and land on her head possibly causing serious injury.

(b) Rotation can be tested in the sitting position by the examiner rotating the shoulders to the limit first in one direction and then in the other. This movement takes place largely at the thoraco-lumbar junction. The average range is about 90 degrees to either side. Because of the third law of spinal movement, it is most important that the patient should sit erect when motion testing is being performed.

(c) Upper thoracic spine—
Screening of movement in this region is most easily done by side bending. There are various methods. The following is the author's preference. (Fig. 7)
1 The patient sits with the legs over the side of the examination table.
2 You stand behind her.
3 Place your right forearm across the patient's right shoulder with the hand resting on the base of the neck and to the left side. The index finger of your right hand points

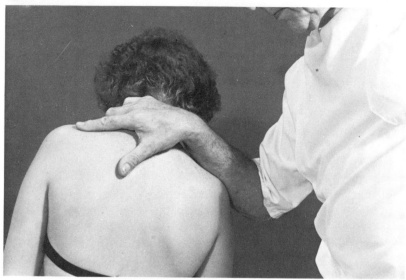

Fig. 7 Screening test for the Thoracic spine.

towards her left shoulder lying on the trapezius muscle, your thumb points down the back and assists in control, your three lateral fingers are curled round the base of the neck.

4 Test by alternately pressing down on the patient's right shoulder and then releasing the pressure and easing the trunk upright again.

5 Monitor with the thumb and index finger of the left hand at the interspinous intervals.

6 If desired repeat the test with the hands reversed.

(d) Overall movement in the cervical spine is also tested in the sitting position with the patient erect. In a normal cervical spine extension ought to be about 90 degrees, flexion of the skull on the neck 45 degrees, and total flexion when the neck is allowed to bend, 90 degrees. Rotation is normally about 90 degrees to either side. Side bending ought to be 45 degrees to either side.

Supine Examination

(a) Note any apparent difference in leg length by comparing the levels of the medial malleoli.

(b) Test the range of movement in the hip and knee joints and note any restriction.

(c) Test for abnormal tightness in the hip muscles especially the hamstrings, the adductors and abductors, and the pyriformis.

When the hamstrings are tighter on one side than the other, stretching by isometric contraction will permit a reassessment of the standing forward flexion test (see page 49).

(d) Height of pubis—this examination is conveniently done at this point although it is not part of the screening. (See Detailed Examination, The Pelvis.)

From the results of the screening examination it is often possible to find pointers to levels which might otherwise be neglected in the detailed examination. For instance, in a patient with almost normal straight leg raising but gross restriction of standing forward flexion, the lower thoracic and thoraco-lumbar joints should always be examined. Unilateral restricted internal rotation of the hip in the 90 degree flexed position (from a tight pyriformis muscle) is often associated with a problem in the sacro-iliac joint on the same side. Restriction of shoulder movement should alert one to examine in detail the cervical and upper thoracic spine.

It should be noted that restriction of movement in one hip joint does not necessarily indicate disease of that joint, particularly if that is the side of the back pain and sciatica. A steel worker in his thirties was seen with pain in the right hip and leg. He had already had several x-rays of the hip which had all been normal. He was unable to flex the hip more than 45 degrees from the extended position and all other movements were restricted. He was sent to the author in the hope that the condition might bear some relation to his previous back trouble. After only one manipulation of the lumbar spine he had improved and in time he regained a full range of hip motion, being treated by spinal manipulation only. Presumably the restriction was due to muscle spasm although clinically it was indistinguishable from that found in severe osteoarthritis. (See also appendix, cases 10 and 11.)

Estimation of Leg Length

The importance of a structural difference in the length of the legs is often overlooked. Even more common is failure to realise that estimation of relative leg length is difficult by any clinical test. The standard measurement from the anterior superior spine to the tip of the medial malleolus is open to gross errors if, as is so common, there is twisting of the pelvis.

Measurement from the greater trochanter to the lateral malleolus is incomplete and tends to be inaccurate, especially in the obese. The clinical methods of estimation which are most helpful are:

1 Comparison of the levels of the posterior superior spines from behind with the patient standing. This is most easily done by finding the posterior superior spines from below with the tips of your thumbs and observing their relative heights (Fig. 8);

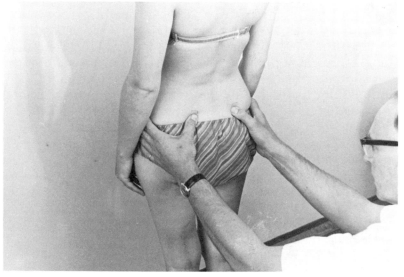

Fig. 8 Estimation of height of posterior iliac spine with the help of the thumbs.

2 Comparison of the height of the posterior superior spines from behind with the patient fully flexed so that you can "sight along" the back and see which side is the higher (Fig. 9);
3 By observing the relative level of the gluteal folds from behind with the patient erect;
4 By comparing the relative height of the two iliac crests with the index finger placed horizontally along the crest (Fig. 10). In this it is easy to be misled by including a thicker layer of soft tissue on one side than on the other. This error is much more likely if the patient has a scoliosis.

In all estimation of heights, it is useful to be aware of one's proprioceptive input in addition to sighting.

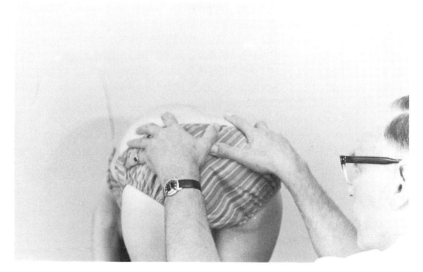

Fig. 9 Estimation of leg length by sighting along the fingers over the posterior spines.

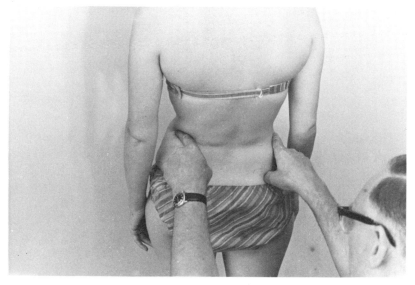

Fig. 10 Estimation of leg length by the fingers on the iliac crests. (The model had lift under the left foot when Figs. 8, 9 and 10 were taken.)

Dr. James Fisk has pointed out that an error can be introduced by having the patient positioned with the heels together. This error is relatively small, but can be important when there is marked unilateral spasm in the low lumbar or gluteal muscles. If, owing to such muscle spasm, the patient is standing with the weight more on one side than the other and leaning toward that side, there will be a slight apparent increase in the length of the leg away from which the patient leans, because the heels are closer together than the hip joints. If the heels are placed about six inches apart, a parallelogram is formed, the base being the floor and the sides being the lines joining the heels to the centre of movement of the hip joints. Simple geometry tells us that the relative height of the hip joints must then remain the same even if the angle made between the side and the base is changed (Fig. 11).

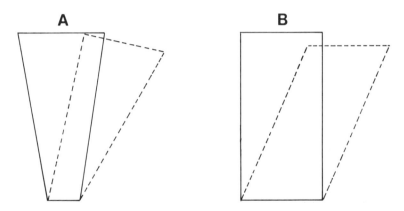

Fig. 11 Diagram to show the possible error in estimation of leg length if the feet are close together.

If there is suspicion of a difference in leg length, the patient should next be seated on the table with the legs over the side. You stand behind her and again estimate the relative height of the posterior inferior spines (Fig. 12). With the patient sitting the effect of any leg length discrepancy is eliminated. If, therefore, the right posterior superior spine is lower than the left with the patient standing, but level with the patient sitting, there is evidence that the right leg is shorter than the left. If, with the patient sitting, the posterior superior spine on the right still appears lower than that on the left, the probable cause is a fixed torsion of the pelvis.

In some patients it is possible to distinguish between the short leg and pelvic torsion by examination from the front with the patient standing. If the anterior and posterior spines are higher on the same side, a difference in leg length is indicated. If on

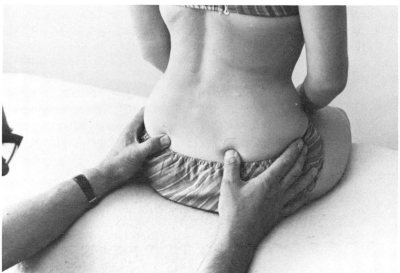

Fig. 12 Sitting estimation of height of posterior spines.

opposite sides, there is likely to be pelvic torsion. The possibility of observer error in these estimations must always be remembered.

Detailed Examination
THE PELVIS
It is helpful to consider the body in the supine position first. The sacrum is now stabilized between the ilia. If the pelvis twists, one ilium will rotate posteriorly with respect to the sacrum; the other will rotate anteriorly. The sulcus between the posterior superior iliac spine and the sacrum will become deep on the side of the posterior innominate, and that on the other side shallow. The symphysis will undergo torsion without translation.

Now turn the body over. The ilia are now supported by the table. The sacrum can flex and extend but it can also twist about an oblique axis extending roughly from the superior pole of one articular surface to the inferior pole of the other. The left axis is the one starting at the left superior pole. Torsion can occur about either oblique axis and in either direction on that axis. This torsion must, of course, be associated with one innominate being posterior and the other anterior with respect to the sacrum. Unfortunately, the complexity is such that the result is not precisely the same when the sacral torsion is primary as it is when the iliac displacement is primary. Either can occur and the treatment is not always the same.

The most important diagnostic points in the assessment of pelvic dysfunction are:

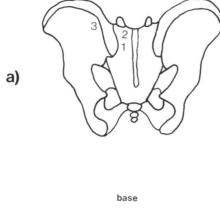

a)

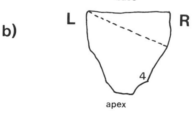

b)

base

L   R

4

apex

Fig. 13 (a) Articulated pelvis from behind. For meaning of figures see text. (b) Diagram of sacrum from behind. Dotted line marks the left oblique axis. 4 marks the right inferior lateral angle.

1 The inferior lateral angle (ILA) of the sacrum. (Fig. 13(b) 4)
2 The sulcus between the PSIS and the back of the sacrum. (Fig. 13(a) 1–2)
3 The relative level of the pubic bone on either side.
4 The apparent change in leg length due to asymmetry in the position of the ilia.
5 The depth of the lumbar lordosis.

The ILA is found directly lateral to the sacral cornua about three-quarters of an inch from the midline.

Apparent differences in leg length are observed by comparing the levels of the medial malleoli.

The disturbances of the sacrum between the ilia can be classified as follows:

1 Unilateral Sacral Flexion—The sacrum will not extend on the ilium on one side. On the side that is restricted the sulcus between the PSIS and the sacrum will be deep and the inferior lateral angle will be inferior and slightly posterior compared to the other side.

2 Forward Sacral Torsion (as with vertebrae the direction of rotation is described by the way the anterior surface of the sacrum turns)—In this case the sacrum turns to the same side as the axis on which it is turning. The torsion may be to the left on the left oblique axis or to the right on the right axis.

3 Backward Sacral Torsion—Either to the right on the left axis or to the left on the right axis.

Sacral torsions are diagnosed by:

1 Loss of movement at the sacro-iliac joint.
2 A deep sulcus on one side.
3 The ILA is relatively posterior (and slightly inferior) on the opposite side to the deep sulcus.
4 An apparent short leg in the prone position on the opposite side to the deep sulcus.
5 Forward and backward sacral torsions are distinguished by the depth of the lumbar lordosis.

A deep sulcus on the right and a posterior ILA on the left may signify forward torsion on the left (Lt on Lt) or backward torsion on the right axis (Lt on Rt). In order to distinguish between them use is made of the fact that in forward torsion the sacrum is slightly flexed and in backward torsion slightly extended. The position of the sacrum of course affects that of the lumbar spine. In forward torsion there will be a slight increase in lordosis. The lordosis can be tested by springing the lumbar spine in the prone position. If it springs easily it indicates lordosis (and therefore a forward torsion). If it feels rigid and does not spring easily it indicates a backward torsion.

As a confirmation of the lumbar springing test the backward bending test can be used. In backward bending the positional changes in a backward torsion are exaggerated while those in a forward torsion are diminished. The pelvis should be re-examined with the patient still prone but the spine extended by having her "get up on her elbows" supporting the chin in the hands. If the positional changes are now difficult to find, the torsion was forward. If the positional changes are exaggerated, the torsion was backward.

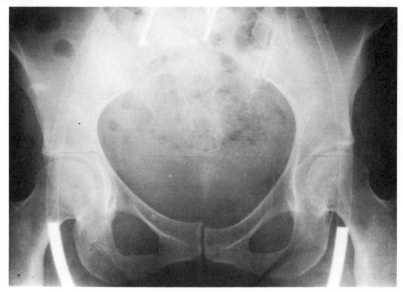

Fig. 14 Standing x-ray of pelvis showing asymmetry of the pubic symphysis. The plastic tube hoop, half filled with radio-opaque fluid, enables one to draw a true horizontal on the film in order to measure leg length differences.

Subluxation of the Symphysis Pubis (Fig. 14)

Subluxation is a proper term for what is an abnormal movement. This can be detected by comparing the height of the pubic bones on either side of the symphysis. The index finger of either hand is hooked over the superior aspect of the pubic bone one half to one inch lateral to the symphysis. Care must be taken to avoid having one finger on the pubic tubercle when that on the other side is on the body of the bone. The side to be considered abnormal is that on which the standing flexion test was positive at the sacro-iliac joint.

In earlier editions other methods of estimating motion at the sacro-iliac joints were described and they are included briefly for those who may wish to use them instead of, or in addition to, the flexion tests.

The Leg Lengthening Test

1 The patient lies supine.
2 To eliminate chance asymmetry of position she places her feet on the top of the couch, lifts up her pelvis and then puts it down again.

3 The legs are then extended and allowed to lie on the table.
4 Note the relative position of the medial malleoli.
5 You pick up first one leg and then the other and perform similar movements.
6 The circumduction which will shorten the leg (where the sacro-iliac joint is mobile) is performed by flexion of the knee and hip in abduction, bringing the thigh up through full flexion in the neutral position and then through internal rotation in adduction to the starting position on the couch (Fig. 15). No jerk is required.

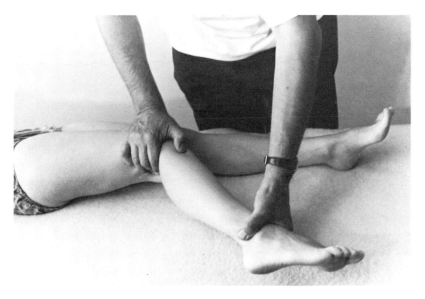

Fig. 15 The leg shortening manoeuvre.

7 The reverse movement, flexion through the adducted internally rotated position, to full flexion, to abduction in external rotation and then back to the couch produces lengthening (Fig. 16).

NOTE:
    (1) The amount of lengthening and shortening with normal mobility is about half an inch in each direction.
    (2) The increase or decrease in apparent leg length is due to alteration in the vertical height (in the anatomical position) of the sacral base above the hip joint which occurs secondarily to sacro-iliac angular movement.

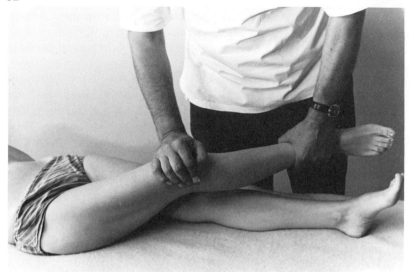

Fig. 16 The leg lengthening manoeuvre for testing sacro-iliac mobility.

When the hip is extended so that the long axis of the thigh is parallel to that of the trunk, Brooke's centre of movement lies behind the long axis of the thigh. (See Fig. 1, Ch. 2) An angle is formed between the lines A–B and B–C, A being the centre of movement of the sacro-iliac joint, B being the centre of movement of the hip joint, and C being a point vertically below B at the surface of the floor on which the foot is standing. The effective length of the limb is dependent on the length of the line A–D rather than that of the line B–C, D being a point on the floor vertically below the point A. If the innominate bone is rotated forward relative to the sacrum the angle θ is increased and therefore the length of the line A–D is increased, giving an apparently lengthening of the limb. Similarly, if the innominate is rotated backwards the angle θ and therefore the length of the line A–D is decreased.

Prone Springing Test

1 The patient lies prone.
2 You stand to her left side.
3 With your elbow straight you apply springing pressure with the heel of your right hand on the apex of her sacrum.
4 Monitor movement with your left thumb in the sulcus between the sacrum and the posterior superior iliac spine on both sides

(Fig. 17). Patients with sacro-iliac strains will often complain of localized pain when this movement is performed.

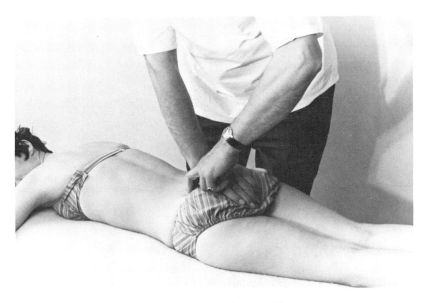

Fig. 17 Sacral springing to test sacro-iliac mobility.

Supine Flexion Test

1 The patient lies supine.
2 To examine the right side you stand to her right.
3 You flex her right knee and hip fully and control the limb by holding the knee in your axilla and with your right hand.
4 With your left hand palpate her right sacro-iliac region, sliding the hand under her buttock so that the terminal and middle phalanges of the index and the middle fingers span the gap between the sacrum and posterior superior spine.
5 Lock the femur against the ilium by full adduction and flexion.
6 Rock the ilium on the sacrum by alternately increasing and decreasing the flexion and adduction of the thigh, monitoring movement with your left hand (Fig. 18).

NOTE:

The stability of the left side of the pelvis can be increased by allowing the patient's left leg and thigh to hang over the opposite side of the table.

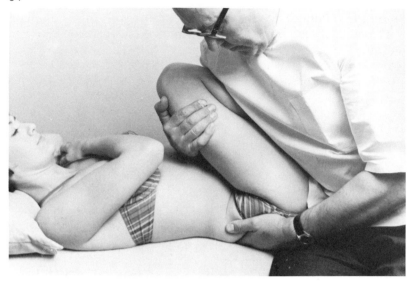

Fig. 18 Rocking the ilium to test sacro-iliac mobility.

Tenderness and Muscle Tension in Pelvis

As has already been mentioned, there is no convenient muscle in which excess tension is diagnostic of sacro-iliac strain. Unilateral increased tension is usually found in the lower part of the erector spinae. There is, however, a characteristic point of tenderness which can be found in nearly all cases that have symptoms. This point lies at the lower end of the sulcus, to the medial side of the posterior superior spine, between it and the spinous processes of the first and second sacral vertebrae (Fig. 13(a) 1). It is important that the site of this point should be appreciated because there are other tender spots in the neighbourhood which do not necessarily point to the sacro-iliac joint. The first of these is between the posterior superior iliac spine and that of the 5th lumbar vertebra (Fig. 13(a) 2). This is the most common site of tenderness in a lumbosacral joint dysfunction. The second is in the origin of the gluteal muscles immediately lateral to the posterior iliac spines (Fig. 13(a) 3). The latter point is very commonly tender in patients with low back pain. The joint lesion which causes the formation of this tender spot may be found from as far up as the low thoracic region down to the sacro-iliac joint itself. In patients with joint lesions low down, the maximum tenderness is usually found low down but in those with higher lesions, the maximum tenderness may be found more laterally below the iliac crest.

This tenderness is associated with a palpable thickening in the muscle. For many years the term "fibrositis" was used for this condition and when so used was useful. It has now fallen into disrepute because of a failure to distinguish the various causes of pain in the back.

The examination of the point of tenderness for the sacro-iliac joint can be done either with the patient prone or rather more easily, with the patient in the lateral position and the hip flexed.

THE LUMBAR SPINE

Spinal joints are examined to determine their mobility, the position at which movement is restricted and the presence or absence of abnormal muscle tension. Information leading to the establishment of a reasonably precise diagnosis can be obtained by the two findings of loss of motion and localized abnormal muscle tension. Full diagnosis depends on the determination of precisely where, in its range, the movement of the joint is restricted.

For many years the author used stiffness and muscle tension alone as guides to treatment and some will find this approach easier. It has certain disadvantages, however, and the author recommends that even if one starts that way, one should progress to positional diagnosis.

Motion and Muscle Tension Testing

In previous editions of this book positional diagnosis was not discussed. A technique by which one can determine movement and muscle tension abnormalities was described and is included here. All these techniques require training of the fingers and the brain to appreciate small differences in tension as well as other changes. From these observations one often obtains useful information about position.

1 For examination of the left side of the spine, the patient lies on her right.
2 You stand in front of her.
3 Persuade her to relax. To assist this her head should be supported either by her right arm or by a pillow.
4 Her right shoulder should be pulled slightly forwards because it is easier to control the movement if the coronal plane of her body is tilted back from the vertical.
5 Grasp her left leg and flex the hip and knee.

6 Control the position of the left leg either with your right hand (Fig. 19) or your abdomen (Fig. 20).

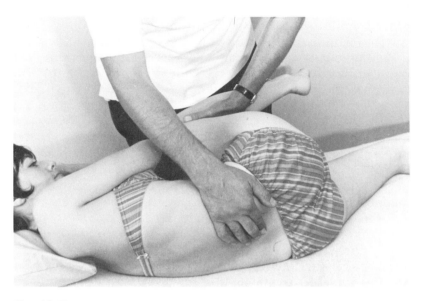

Fig. 19 Testing individual lumbar mobility.

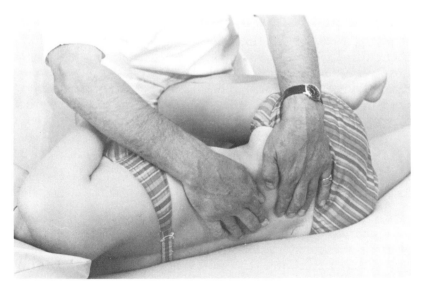

Fig. 20 Testing individual lumbar mobility with both hands.

7 By moving sideways you can flex and extend the lumbar spine at the level under examination.

8 Monitor movement at each interspinous interval in turn using the index and middle or better the two index fingertips.

9 Using the same movement examine the left lateral musculature for abnormal tension at each level.

10 Turn the patient over and repeat the examination from the other side.

NOTE:

(1) If the patient is lying in the correct position it is relatively easy to use your abdomen to control the movement of her thigh. When this can be done it permits the use of the two index fingers for palpation.

(2) It is easier to monitor two interspinous intervals at the same time in order to compare the range of movement.

(3) The greater the flexion of the hip, the higher up in the lumbar spine is the movement produced.

(4) No attempt should be made to estimate abnormal muscle tension on the side on which the patient is lying. This examination is unreliable.

(5) The whole of the lumbar spine and the lowest part of the thoracic region can be tested by this procedure.

In order to compare the muscle tension on the two sides without moving the patient the prone position must be used but, below the fourth lumbar vertebra, it is essential that the spine should be flexed. This may be done either by having the patient lie across the table with the hips well flexed, or by having her in the "knee-elbow" position.

Position Testing

(A) Static

1 The patient lies prone.

2 You stand to either side and palpate the transverse processes of each vertebra in turn with your thumbs. The transverse process in the lumbar spine is found lateral to the longissimus muscle, about 1 to $1\frac{1}{4}$ inch from the midline.

3 The object is to assess the relative position of the two transverse processes in the anteroposterior (sagittal) plane.

4 With the thumbs on the transverse processes it is an advantage to sight nearly horizontally in order to observe whether one is more posterior than the other.

5 Note which vertebrae are rotated with one transverse process more posterior than the other. Note in which direction they are rotated (that is, which is the most posterior of the rotated transverse processes).

6 Repeat the examination with the lumbar spine in flexion. This can be done either in the same position as the seated flexion test for sacro-iliac movement, or in the knee-elbow position on the table.

7 Repeat the examination with the spine in extension. This is achieved by having the patient support her head in her hands, with the elbows together and resting on the table directly under the shoulders. The patient must be encouraged to relax or the abdominal muscles may prevent proper hyperextension.

NOTE:

(1) If only one vertebra is rotated it is likely to be a type II lesion. In this case the position will be exaggerated in either flexion or extension as compared to neutral. It should be treated in the position which aggravates the deformity.

(2) If more than one vertebra is found to be rotated it is probably a compensatory type I lesion and in that case the vertebra at the apex of the curve should be treated in the neutral position.

(B) Dynamic

The position of the lumbar vertebrae can also be assessed by the test described (Ch. 4, p. 73) for the thoracic spine.

REFERENCES

1 Kimberely, P. E. (1980), Formulating a Prescription for Osteopathic Manipulative Treatment, *JAOA* **79**, 506–513.

2 Mennell, J. M. (1975), The Therapeutic use of Cold, *JAOA* **74**, 1146–1158.

4

Examination

The Thoracic Spine
The Ribs
The Cervical Spine
X-rays

THE THORACIC SPINE

Motion Testing

This is done with the patient sitting and, because of the third law of spinal movement, she should sit erect.

There are a variety of methods.

(A) Sitting test for T3–T11 (Fig. 21):

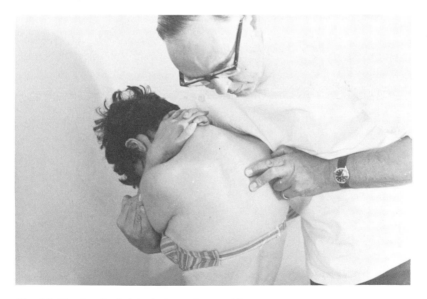

Fig. 21 Testing individual thoracic mobility.

1   The patient sits with her legs over the side of the table.
2   You stand behind her.
3   Have her lace her hands behind her neck and allow her elbows to fall together in front. Grasp her elbows with one hand and induce flexion and extension in the thoracic spine by lifting and lowering them. In those with shoulder stiffness an alternative grip may be necessary.
3a You hook your right arm under her right axilla and place your right hand on the back of the lower neck. Stability can be increased by having the patient put her right hand on the back of her head (Fig. 22); or,

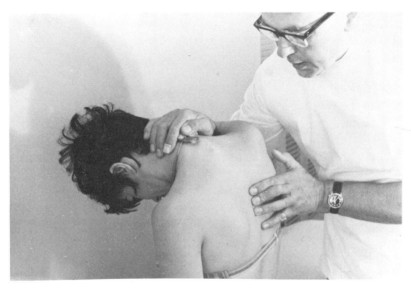

Fig. 22 Testing individual thoracic mobility in presence of a stiff left shoulder joint.

3b You hook your right arm under her right axilla and pass the hand across the front of the chest to grip her left shoulder. Stability in this position is increased by the patient taking hold of her right shoulder with her left hand.
4   With your other hand, monitor the movement at each joint in turn. The index and middle fingers are used to palpate the interspinous ligaments.
(B) Sitting test for lower cervical and upper thoracic joints (Fig. 23):

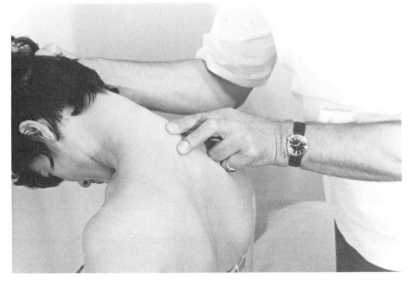

Fig. 23 Testing individual mobility in the upper thoracic joints.

    1 The patient sits with her legs over the side of the table.
    2 You stand behind her.
    3 You grasp her head with one hand and induce movement
      by flexion and extension of the head and neck.
    4 With your other hand you monitor movement at each
      interspinous interval in turn.
(C) To test side bending and rotation either of the alternative
    grips described under (A) 3a or 3b may be used. The
    movement is monitored by your other hand at each joint
    in turn (Fig. 24).
(D) Mobility can also be tested in the prone position (Fig. 25):
    1 The patient lies prone and relaxed.
    2 You stand beside her.
    3 With a downward springing pressure by one or both
      hands the mobility of each segment can be tested.
    4 The pressure should be applied over the spinous process
      at each level in turn. The pressure should be momentary
      and light. It is not desirable to perform an extension
      manipulation at this stage.
NOTE:
    (1) It is an advantage if the table is low enough for the arms
        to be nearly straight.
    (2) The pressure should be almost directly downwards
        (towards the anterior aspect of the patient's body).

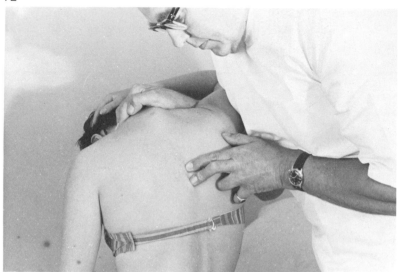

Fig. 24 Testing individual joint rotation in the thoracic region.

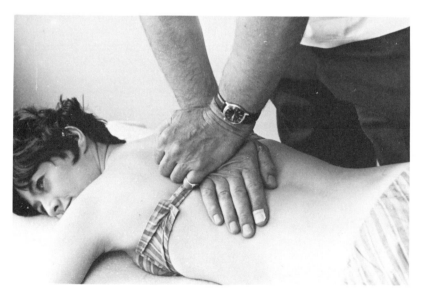

Fig. 25 "Springing" the thoracic spine.

(3) If pain and muscle spasm is produced by this test performed gently, it should alert you to the possibility of a destructive lesion at this level rather than a simple somatic dysfunction.

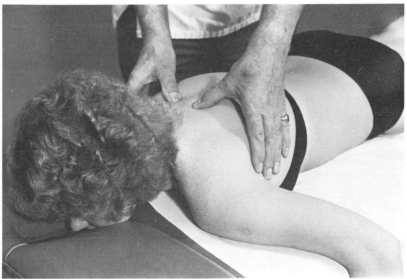

Fig. 26 Static position testing in the thoracic spine. Note the slot in the table allowing the head to rest centrally. The examiner's master eye should be over the patient's midline. It may be necessary to stoop to be sure which of the thumbs is the most posterior.

Position Testing
(A) Static (Fig. 26)
    1 The patient lies prone.
    2 You stand to either side, preferably with your master eye over the patient's midline.
    3 Palpate the transverse processes of each vertebra in turn with your thumbs noting which is the most posterior (as in the test described for the lumbar spine).

NOTE:
    (1) In the thoracic spine it is important that the head should be central and not turned to one side. A table or a cushion with a slot to accommodate nose and chin is helpful.
    (2) In the thoracic spine the transverse processes are closer together than in the lumbar region. The tip of the transverse process lies about seven-eighths to one inch from the midline.

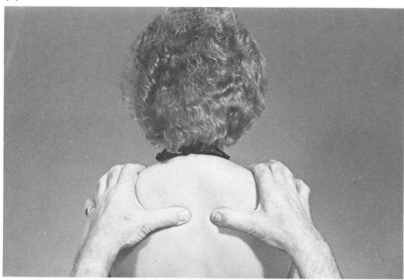

(a)

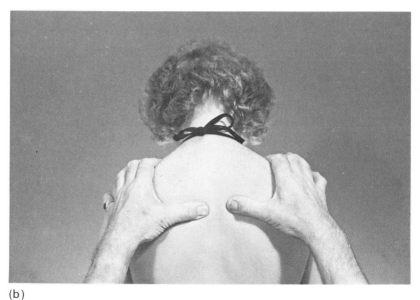

(b)

Fig. 27 Dynamic position testing in the thoracic spine. (a) Thumbs placed on transverse processes of T3 in neutral flexion. (b) In forward flexion of this area the right thumb rides up but the left remains down and more prominent (indicating failure of the left facet joint to open). (c) In extension the thumbs ride down and back equally.

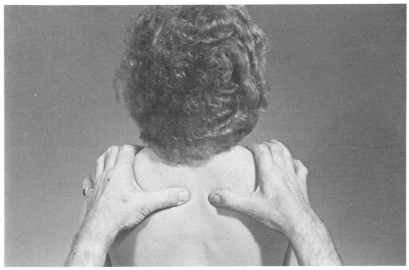

(c)

(B) Dynamic (Fig. 27)

 1 The patient sits erect with the spine in "neutral". For the
   upper thoracic joints, sitting with the legs over the side
   of the examination table will do. For the lower joints and
   for the lumbar spine a suitable stool is better. If the table
   is used, the feet should be supported.
 2 You stand behind the patient with your master eye
   behind her midline.
 3 With your thumbs palpate the two transverse processes or
   facets of each vertebra in turn. It need hardly be added
   that it is only necessary to perform these tests in areas
   where the screening examination has shown an abnormality.
 4 The patient flexes the head and neck fully. You observe
   whether the movement of the transverse processes (or
   facets) is equal.
 5 The patient then extends fully—the same observation is
   made. The movements need to be fairly slow and for
   levels below about T5 the trunk must be flexed as well
   as the neck and head. Hence the need to support her feet.

NOTE:

 (1) It will be found that a transverse process or facet that
   does not flex remains prominent under the thumb. The
   normal moves forward and is felt less easily. Corres-

pondingly a facet or transverse process that will not extend remains forward and difficult to feel. The moving side becomes more prominent in extension.

(2) In patients with group dysfunction following Type I mechanics the facet movement is different. It will usually be found that both facets will extend fully and will flex fully but that in the mid range (neutral) there is a differential movement in which if the left facet fails to open as soon as the right, the *right* side will feel more prominent. This corresponds to the Type I (neutral) mechanics in which sidebending and rotation are to opposite sides.

(3) Some patients have difficulty in understanding how to do the movement. If necessary, the examination can be done with the index and middle fingers of one hand while your other hand guides the movement.

From the information obtained by this test both position and movement can be assessed.

(a) If the left transverse process of T3 will not ride up on flexion —but that on the right does ride up—there is restriction of flexion, of right sidebending and of right rotation at the T3–4 joint.

(b) If both transverse processes ride up equally, but the right one will not come back fully, there is restriction of extension, of right sidebending and of right rotation at the joints.

It is easier to understand these movements and their implications if one thinks of the movements of the facets themselves, see Fig. 28.

Muscle Tension Testing

This may be done sitting, prone, or supine.

Sitting

Except for the upper few joints it is difficult to get the patient to relax enough. It is of some value for what may be an unexpected reason. Patients when they first come, are often apprehensive. Lesions in the upper thoracic spine are very common, particularly in those complaining of symptoms in the head, neck and upper trunk. Many patients come to a manipulator after they have been to other practitioners who have failed to find the cause of the problem. This increases their apprehension. If one can demonstrate quickly by palpation that one can find a lesion, the patient will immediately know. Confidence

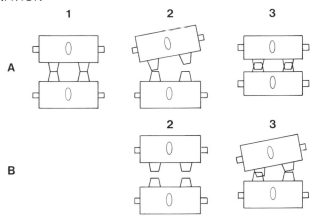

Fig. 28 Diagram to show movement of facets. In column 1 the spine is in neutral. In column 2 the spine is forward flexed. In column 3 the spine is extended. In line A there is restriction of flexion at the left facet joint. This automatically causes left sidebending (and left rotation) of the upper vertebra on the lower. In extension both facet joints close fully. In line B there is normal opening on flexion but the right facet joint fails to close. This also produces left sidebending and left rotation of the upper vertebra on the lower.

is established and the patient will then relax. This materially assists the rest of the examination.

1 The patient sits with the legs over the side of the table.
2 You stand facing her.
3 Rest her head against the front of your chest.
4 Palpate the posterior muscles on either side over the transverse processes.

NOTE:
   (1) It is usually possible to find one or more levels at which the tension is above normal. These areas will be tender and, if you press more firmly, the patient will know at once that you have found something.
   (2) For palpating muscles in the thoracic spine (probably because of its kyphosis) it is often easier to move one's fingers up and down across the transverse process. In the cervical and lumbar regions, it is easier to feel if one makes the movement transversely across the muscle fibres.

Prone
   For the overall assessment of muscle tension in the thoracic region, the prone position is commonly used. It is most important

that the head should be central and not turned to one side. Here again a table with a slot for the nose and chin, or a cushion with such a slot is helpful. The tension in the muscle should be palpated with the pads of the fingers. When an abnormality is found it is important to determine which of the muscle layers is affected. The implication of tension abnormalities in the superficial muscles is quite different. Their innervation is not derived from the underlying joint.

Supine

It is also possible to assess muscle tension with the patient supine. The advantage is that most people relax more easily in the supine position. There is a disadvantage, however. In the supine position it is only possible to feel one side at a time.

1 The patient lies supine.
2 To feel for muscle tension on the patient's left side, you stand at her right.
3 Raise her left shoulder with your left hand and feel the muscles at the upper thoracic levels with the fingers of your right hand.

With this technique it is not easy to feel accurately below about T6.

THE RIBS

Ribs move in two different ways although the movement is, of course, related. On inhalation the sternum rides upwards. In order to achieve this the ribs move so that the front end rises and this is known as pump-handle movement. The main axis of this movement is roughly transverse. Also on inhalation the transverse diameter of the chest increases. This is produced by what is known appropriately as bucket-handle movement. The ribs rotate about an axis which is more or less antero-posterior so that the middle of the rib becomes elevated and everted.[1]

It is clear that there is an element of each movement in the motion of all ribs. The upper ribs have more pump-handle motion while the lower have more of a bucket-handle type.

This description must be modified for the eleventh and twelfth ribs which have no fixed anterior attachment.

Restriction of pump-handle motion is best felt at the anterior end of the rib but bucket-handle restriction will be more obvious in the axilla.

Techniques of examination are not quite the same but the principle is simple. The observation depends on noting restriction of rib movement on inhalation or exhalation.

When there is a restriction, the rib(s) on the affected side can be felt to stop moving before those on the other side. This applies both in inhalation and exhalation. Because of its position, relative to neighbouring normal ribs, a rib with an inhalation restriction is sometimes termed depressed and one with an exhalation restriction elevated.

Ribs move together in normal breathing and a restriction at one level will affect the mobility of the neighbouring ribs. If the first rib has an inhalation restriction it will be physically impossible for the second rib to move up fully. The first will be in the way. Similarly if the fifth rib has an exhalation restriction the fourth will also have limited movement. The ribs further away will have some restriction but the effect tends to diminish.

The importance of this is that when an inhalation restriction is found it is essential to find (and to treat) the uppermost restricted rib. When the restriction is in exhalation the lowest restricted rib is the one to treat first. Following the initial treatment a re-examination will show if other ribs also need to be treated.

Examination for Rib Restriction

1 *Upper Ribs*

(A) Inhalation (Fig. 29)

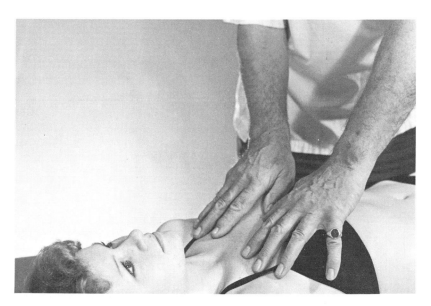

Fig. 29 Position for testing movement in the upper ribs.

1 The patient is supine.

2 You stand to the side which most easily brings your master eye over the midline of her trunk.

3 Place the hands lightly, flat on the front of her chest with the tips of the index fingers just below the inner end of the clavicle and the hands roughly parallel to the sternum.

4 Have her take a deep breath in. Follow the movement with your hands and eyes.

5 If one side has a pump-handle inhalation restriction it will stop moving before the other side.

(B) Exhalation

Steps 1, 2, and 3 as in (A) above.

4 Have the patient take a small breath in and then breathe out to the limit. Follow the movement with your hands and eyes.

5 If one side has a pump-handle exhalation restriction it will stop moving before the other side.

(C) Bucket-Handle Restrictions

Failure of enlargement of the transverse diameter of the upper thorax can be felt in a similar manner but the hands should make an angle of about 45 degrees to the vertical axis of the body. In this way the movement of the axillary part of the rib is more easily felt.

The procedure in other respects is the same as for pump-handle restrictions.

NOTE:

(1) In the upper ribs the normal motion is predominantly pump-handle and restrictions of pump-handle motion are both more common and more important.

(2) The distinction between motion that is of pump-handle type from that which is bucket handle is much less important than the distinction between inhalation and exhalation restriction.

2 *Middle Ribs* (5, 6, 7)

1 The patient is supine.

2 You stand to the side that brings your master eye over her midline.

3 Place your hands lightly on the front of her chest with the thumbs on the sternal end of the fifth costal cartilages and your fingers following the fifth, sixth and seventh ribs.

4 For inhalation restrictions have her take a deep breath in.

For exhalation restrictions she should take a small breath in and then breathe out to the limit.

5 In this position restriction of pump-handle motion can be felt if one thumb stops moving before the other. Restriction of bucket-handle motion is indicated if the fingertips on one side stop moving before the others.

3 *Lower Ribs* (8, 9, 10)

1 The patient is supine.
2 You stand to the side that brings your master eye over her midline.
3 Place your hands lightly over the lower ribs with the thumbs resting along the costal margin and their tips just caudal to the xiphoid process.
4 Perform inhalation and exhalation testing in the same way noting pump-handle restrictions with the thumbs and bucket-handle restrictions with the fingertips.

NOTE:

In the lower ribs bucket-handle movement predominates and restrictions are usually of bucket handle movement.

4 *Floating Ribs* (11, 12)

1 Restrictions here can be detected with the patient prone.
2 You stand to the side that brings your master eye over her midline.
3 Find the twelfth ribs, follow to the tips and monitor for movement with the index fingers on the tips of the twelfth ribs and the middle fingers on the eleventh.
4 Note if on either side movement stops "early" in either inhalation or exhalation.

THE CERVICAL SPINE

Motion Testing

The typical cervical joints C2–C7 can be tested in a manner similar to that used for the thoracic spine.

The atlanto-occipital and atlanto-axial joints are atypical and require an understanding of their different properties. Because there is very little rotation at the atlanto-occipital joint, and because there is no side bending at the atlanto-axial, these movements are used to test for motion.

The second law of spinal motion does not apply normally to typical cervical joints. Rotation can be assumed always to be the concavity of the side bend, except at the atlanto-occipital joint.

Atlanto-Occipital Joint

At this joint side bending is used. Two methods will be described.
(A) 1 The patient lies supine.
    2 You stand or sit at her head supporting it in your hands.
    3 Place the tip of the index finger in the gap between the mastoid process and the lateral mass of the atlas on either side.
    4 Side bend the head to the right and note the opening of the gap on the left side and the closing on the right.
    5 Side bend to the left and compare the ranges of movement.
(B) (Fig. 30)
    1 The patient lies supine.
    2 You stand at her head supporting it in your hands.
    3 With the neck in the neutral position of flexion-extension, you make a translatory movement, first to one side and then to the other.
    4 Compare how far the midline of the head can be moved away from the midline of the body to either side.
    5 Repeat with the neck in full flexion.
    6 Repeat with the neck in full extension.

NOTE:
    (1) If translation to the right is restricted there is loss of side bending to the left.

(a)

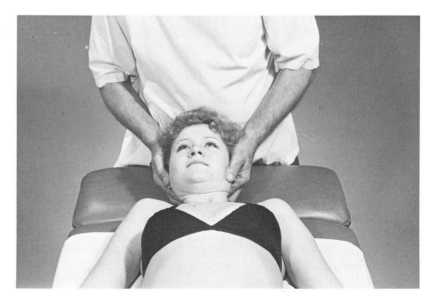

o)

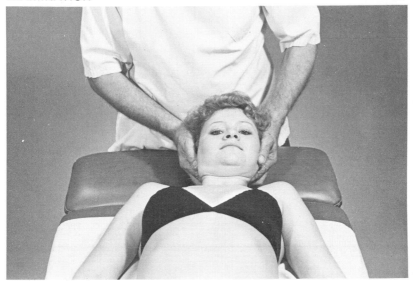

Fig. 30 Testing for sidebending in the atlanto-occipital joint. In (a) the midline of the head has moved more than 1 inch lateral to the mid-line of the body. In (b) the head has not moved so far laterally indicating restriction of right sidebending at the atlanto-occipital joint.

(2) That the flexion-extension position showing the maximum restriction of sidebending is the one to use in treatment.

(3) That restriction of sidebending at joints lower in the neck may affect this test and they should therefore be examined and, if necessary, treated first.

Atlanto-Axial Joint

At this joint rotation is used for testing mobility. Again two methods will be described.

(A) 1 The patient is supine.

2 You stand at her head supporting it in your left hand.

3 Your left thumb is placed in front of the left lateral mass of her atlas.

4 Your left index finger is hooked round the spinous process of the axis to lie on its right side.

5 You hold the chin with your right hand and rotate the head. On rotation of the head to the left the thumb and index finger are approximated, on rotation to the right they move apart.

6 Change your hands. Support the head with your right

hand and use the thumb and index finger to monitor the movement from the other side.

NOTE:
The front of the lateral mass of the atlas is always tender and this tenderness is not a diagnostic sign.

(B) (Fig. 31)
  1 The patient is supine.
  2 You stand at her head holding it in your hands.
  3 You flex the neck fully without flexing the head on the neck.
  4 With both hands you rotate the head, first to the right and then to the left and compare the range of movement.

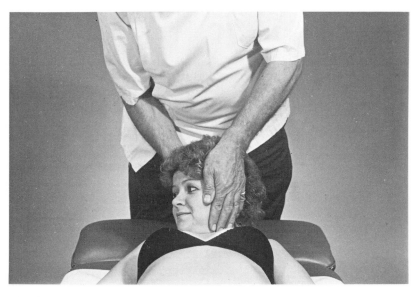

Fig. 31 Testing for movement at the atlanto-axial joint. The range of movement to the right is compared with that to the left.

NOTE:
  (1) The flexion of the rest of the neck almost abolishes rotation below the atlanto-axial joint according to the third law of spinal motion. This law, however, does not apply to the atlanto-axial joint in this position.
  (2) The range of rotation in this position is normally in excess of 60 degrees to either side.

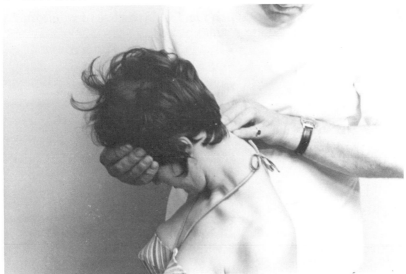

Fig. 32 Testing individual cervical mobility.

The Typical Cervical Joints (C2–C7)

(A) Flexion—Extension (Fig. 32)
  1 The patient sits on a stool or with her legs over the side of the examination table.
  2 You stand behind her.
  3 Grasp her head with your right hand to control its movement.
  4 With the left thumb or index and middle fingers palpate the interspinous intervals.
  5 Rock the head through the appropriate flexion—extension range to cause movement at the joints which are being palpated by the left hand.
  6 Repeat for each joint in turn.

NOTE:
The small size of the posterior tubercle of the atlas and its depth preclude the use of this technique above C2.

(B) Side bending
  1 The patient is supine.
  2 You stand or sit at her head supporting the neck in both hands in neutral flexion.
  3 With the tips of the fingers pressing against the articular pillars of each vertebra in turn, the vertebra is pushed directly sideways (translation).

4 Note any level at which there is restriction of side bending and to which side it will not bend.

5 Repeat with the neck first in flexion and then in extension.

(C) Facet Opening

This technique is similar to that described for the thoracic spine and the same observations apply (see page 73).

1 The patient sits erect or on a suitable stool with her legs over the side of the table.

2 You stand behind her.

3 With the thumbs you palpate the facets on either side at the same level.

4 The patient fully flexes her head and neck.

5 You observe whether one thumb rides up and goes forward more than the other. When a facet rides up it also becomes less prominent on the same side.

6 The patient then extends the head and neck fully.

7 You observe whether both thumbs come down equally.

NOTE:

(1) The movements should be done relatively slowly.

(2) If on flexion one thumb rides up but the other does not, there is a restriction of flexion on the side that does not move.

(3) If on extension one thumb does not come down properly, there is restriction of extension on that side.

(4) If there is a restriction of flexion on the left side, it necessarily follows that that joint must be sidebent and rotated to the side of the flexion restriction. If there is a restriction of extension on the left side, it follows that the restricted joint must be sidebent and rotated to the opposite side.

Position Testing

It will be seen that if motion testing is performed to determine side bending or facet opening, the position of restriction is known. For example, if it is found:

1 That there is resistence to translatory movement to the left at the C4–5 level.

2 That the restriction is greater with the neck flexed than either in neutral or extended, then it can be said that the C4–5 joint has restricted side bending to the right in flexion. We can assume, therefore, that rotation is also restricted to the right.

It is important to recognize the difference between talking of restriction and talking of position. In the above example if one considers the position, the C4–5 joint is sidebent and rotated to the left and extended. In this connection it is an advantage to use a different ending (e.g. Extend*ed*) when talking about the position, to that (e.g. Flex*ion*) used when talking about the direction of motion restriction.

Muscle Tension Testing

(A) (Fig. 33)

    1 The patient lies supine.

    2 The examiner stands at the head of the table.

    3 He supports the head either with his abdomen or with both hands.

    4 The index and middle fingers of both hands feel for muscle tension abnormalities at each level in turn.

This method is preferred for the upper cervical joints down to about C6.

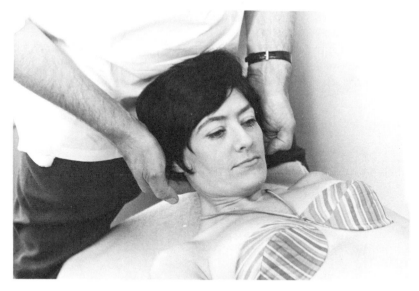

Fig. 33 Feeling the tension in the posterior cervical muscles (supine).

(B) (Fig. 34)

    1 The patient sits on a suitable stool or with the legs over the side of the examination table.

    2 You stand facing her.

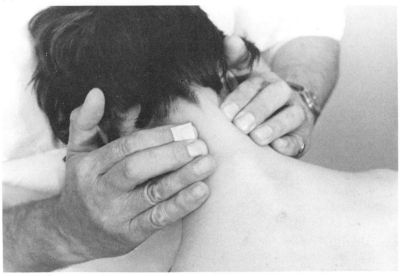

Fig. 34 Feeling the tension in the posterior cervical muscles (sitting).

    3 She rests her head against your chest.
    4 Muscle tension is felt with the index and middle fingers of
      both hands over the back of each joint in turn.
This method is preferred for the lower cervical joints and
can also be used for the upper thoracic spine.

NOTE:
    (1) In the cervical spine the tension is more easily felt by a
        transverse movement of the fingers across the muscle
        rather than the up and down movement recommended
        for the thoracic spine.
    (2) Muscle which is abnormally tight is almost always
        tender.
    (3) Abnormally tight muscle can sometimes be felt to ripple
        as if one were passing one's fingers across a bundle of
        cords.

X-Rays
If one is to rely on x-rays, it is of the utmost importance that
the films are of good quality. Acceptance of evidence from poor
quality films is dangerous. The beginner is very well advised to
see recent x-ray pictures of every spine before he manipulates.
With practice, the manipulator will find that his ability to assess
the condition and the exact position of the vertebrae becomes

good enough to justify confident diagnosis. Then, if one uses techniques of the type described, without anaesthesia and without violence, a single manipulative treatment can be justified in many patients without the precaution of prior radiography. Unfortunately, a negative x-ray is not proof of the absence of a variety of conditions that are better not manipulated. The manipulator must therefore maintain a high index of suspicion for a variety of contraindications. Of these, the most important are osteoporosis, infection, and tumours.

Osteoporosis

Osteoporosis is only common in the comparatively elderly. It is nearly always associated with loss of weight and will always show in an x-ray. If the spinal pain is due to osteoporosis there has already been at least minor collapse of one or more vertebrae even if it does not yet show in the x-rays. On the other hand in many elderly patients with osteoporosis the pain is due to spinal joint dysfunction and will respond to gentle manipulation. In an elderly patient (and the more so if she is losing weight) good x-rays should always be seen before manipulative treatment is started.

Infection

Infection is less important as being both less common and less likely to be missed on clinical grounds. The intensity and widespread nature of the muscle spasm over an infective lesion should immediately put the surgeon on guard and remind him of its possible existence. The fact that the joint cannot be made to move at all by any technique for examination may also arouse his suspicion. The patient is usually ill. The patient with a straight forward back problem is in pain but not ill and the difference can be detected early in most instances. Fortunately the intensity of muscle spasm is sufficient for it to be unlikely that any harm will be done by a single manipulation of the type described in the following chapters, even in a patient with an early infective lesion.

Tumours

The same is not necessarily true of a tumour and although the actual harm that can be done by a single manipulation of a joint in the neighbourhood of a tumour is probably small, this is a danger which must not be forgotten. It is important to remember that bone tumours do not always show in the x-rays even when they are big enough to weaken the structure of the vertebral body.

When x-ray pictures have been taken before the patient is seen for the first time, it is often sufficient to make use of them. If, however, radiography is being undertaken for the purpose, certain special views can be obtained which are of assistance. In the lumbar region it is always desirable to have the standard AP and lateral pictures with obliques to show the integrity of the pedicles and the condition of the facet joints. An antero-posterior picture of the pelvis taken with the patient standing erect, heels on the ground and knees straight, is of great value in assessing any difference in the actual length of the legs (Fig. 35).

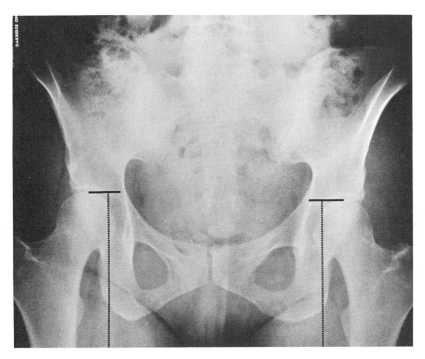

Fig. 35 X-ray showing a structural difference in leg length.

For the examination to be accurate, care must be taken to ensure that the edge of the cassette lies parallel to the floor, or, because this is difficult, to incorporate a marker on the film. This has often been done by a radio-opaque plumb line suspended in front of the film. A simpler and more accurate method has been devised by Dr. Colin Harrison of Vancouver. This does not suffer from the disadvantage of a plumb line which must be allowed to hang free.

Dr. Harrison's method is to use a closed hoop of plastic tubing half filled with a radio-opaque fluid. The hoop is attached by adhesive tape to the x-ray table in such a position that the fluid meniscus on either side is somewhere near the level of the hip joints. A pencil line on the film joining the shadow of the two menisci gives an accurate level. From this line any difference in the height of the hip joints can be measured with a ruler and simple subtraction. Other methods of measuring the length of legs by x-rays are available and are probably more accurate. This method has the advantage of simplicity and of providing a "functional" picture of the pelvis, that is to say, one taken during weight bearing.

If there is gross pelvic torsion this can be seen by one of a variety of changes (Fig. 14).

1 The body of the pubic bone on one side of the symphysis lies higher than that on the other.
2 The outline of the obturator foramen is not symmetrical on the two sides.
3 The shape of the projection of the ilium is different on the two sides.
4 There is a sideways tilting of the sacrum.

As long ago as 1932 Chamberlain[2] described a special technique for x-raying the sacro-iliac joint to demonstrate "sacro-iliac slip". The author does not use this technique but it could prove a convincing demonstration of sacro-iliac mobility, for those who still doubt.

If desired, additional lateral pictures of the lumbar spine can be taken with the spine fully flexed and fully extended. By comparison of these it is possible to confirm the presence of joint stiffness.

In examination of the x-ray film it is of interest to note any deviation of the spinous process of one vertebra from the midline (Figs. 36, 37). The most accurate assessment is made by comparing the distance from the centre of the spinous process to the medial edge of the pedicle on either side. If there is a general deviation of a group of processes in one region, it indicates a Type I lesion. That is a lesion of the type that occurs with the spine in neutral where rotation is to the convexity of the side bend curve. Treatment of these should be done in the neutral position. The finding of a single spinous process deviated to the

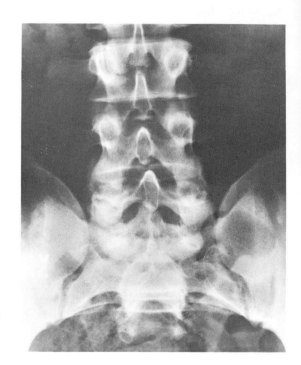

Fig. 36 Deviation of spinous process of L4 to the left side.

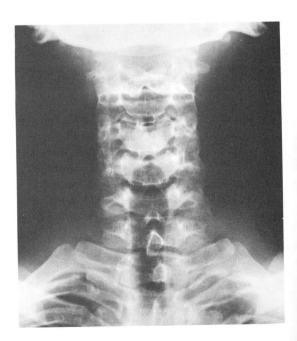

Fig. 37 Deviation of spinous process of T1 to right side.

(a)

(b)

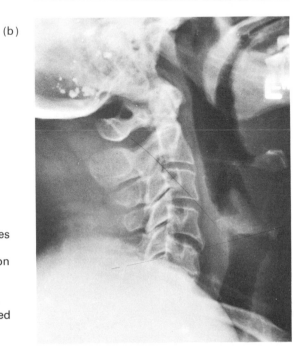

Fig. 38 Cervical
spine showing
degenerative changes
at C4, 5, 6, 7;
comparison of flexion
(a) and extension
(b) views shows
immobility of C2–3
as well as generalised
diminished
movement.

(a)

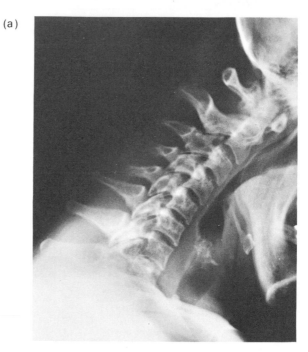

(c)

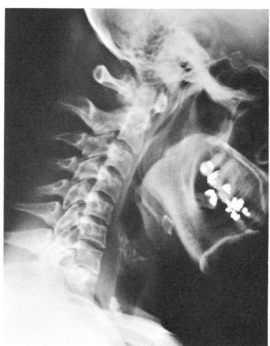

Fig. 39 The three lateral x-ray views of the cervical spine. There is diminished mobility at the atlanto-occipital joint; (a) full flexion, (b) full extension and (c) head flexion ("chin tucked in").

(b)

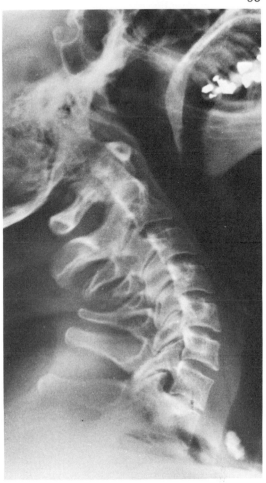

convexity of a short lateral curve (i.e. with the body rotated into the concavity) indicates a Type II lesion occurring either in flexion or extension. These lesions are nearly always traumatic and should be treated first.

In addition to the standard projections for the cervical spine, lateral pictures taken in three additional positions are helpful. If these lateral views are to be taken, the standard lateral can be omitted. These positions are full flexion, full extension and partial neck flexion with the head fully flexed on the neck, the chin being tucked well in. From a comparison of the fully flexed and fully extended pictures it is possible to assess the range of movement in the joints between the vertebrae (Fig. 38). The

(a)

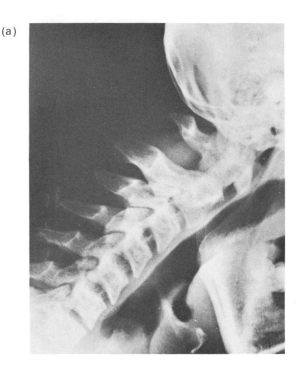

(b)

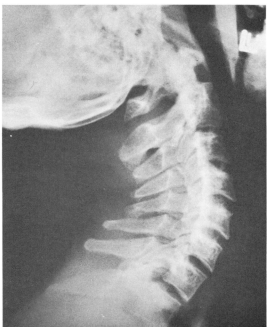

Fig. 40 Three lateral views demonstrating mobility at the atlanto-occipital joints: (a) Full flexion (b) Full extension— note absence of demonstrable movement at C0–1 (c) Head flexion showing opening of gap between occiput and arch of atlas.

(c)

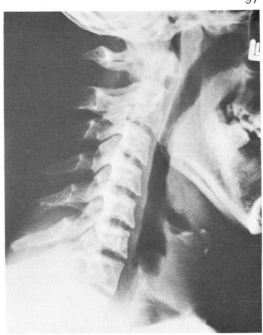

additional film with the chin tucked in is required for assessment
of movement at the atlanto-occipital joint (Figs. 39, 40). In
full flexion of the neck there tends to be some unfolding of the
head, in order to get the chin out of the way, and therefore the
atlanto-occipital joint is not in full flexion. This joint may appear
stiff when the full flexion film is compared with that in full
extension, but its mobility may still be demonstrated by the
third film.

It must be remembered that in the cervical spine the spinous
processes are not usually symmetrical. Assessment of rotation
by the position of the spinous process therefore is not reliable
in the cervical spine except below the C5 vertebra. Details of
techniques for estimating the actual movement at the individual
joints are given by Penning[3].

REFERENCES

1 Kapandji, I. A. (1974), *The Physiology of the Joints*, 2nd Ed., III, 138–143.
  Churchill Livingstone.
2 Chamberlain, W. E. (1932), The X-ray examination of the sacro-iliac joint,
  Delaware State Medical Journal **4**, 195–201.
3 Penning, L. (1968), *Functional Pathology of the Cervical Spine*. Excerpta
  Medica Foundation, Amsterdam.

5

Manipulation

There is at the present time disagreement as to the breadth of meaning of the word manipulation. In Europe the term is reserved almost entirely for procedures involving a high velocity, thrusting movement. In North America it is used in a much wider sense, to include any active or passive movement initiated, assisted or resisted by the physician. This includes treatment sometimes listed as articulation or mobilization, isometric and isotonic contraction techniques and even the so-called functional or indirect techniques where no force at all is applied by the physician.

In the Shorter Oxford English dictionary (second edition, 1939) manipulation is defined in part as: (3) "The handling of objects for a particular purpose; in surgery the manual examination of a part of the body. Also, manual action." There does not appear to be any justification, in the English language at least, for the narrow interpretation of the word and in this volume it will be used in the wide sense.

Types of Manipulation

Many different techniques have been used to alter or remove the restrictive barrier and its associated abnormal muscle tension. In previous editions of this book only high velocity thrusting techniques were described. Non-specific methods were included, but because it is now the author's belief that these should not be regarded even as second best, they have been omitted.

Specific, high velocity techniques are the great standby and have been in use for more than a hundred years. Unfortunately however, they are not without disadvantage and, occasionally, hazard.

Techniques which do not involve the application of anything other than resistive external force have advantages. This is especially true in the aged, in the osteoporotic, in those in whom the pain is too severe to permit a thrusting procedure and in those who are sick (if for any reason it is thought advisable to treat an area of somatic dysfunction at that time).

High Velocity Manipulation

In this method the lesion is diagnosed. The location of the pathological barrier is found and, by a combination of positioning and application of external force, the joint is pushed through the barrier. Obviously the force must be controlled so that it does not push the joint beyond the anatomical barrier or damage will result. This is one of the difficulties. The amount of movement required is small and the force needed may be considerable. It is always difficult to stop a considerable force after only a small distance.

The lever principle can be used with advantage. If it is possible to apply the force through a long lever, the strength of the force is divided, and the distance travelled is multiplied by the ratio of the length of the long lever to that of the shorter one. The application of this will be discussed in descriptions of actual high velocity treatments.

Mobilisation or Articulation

In this method the barrier is once again found but this time, instead of forcing the joint through it, the barrier is almost caressed. By taking the joint gently up to the barrier, moving beside (if such movement is available) and then away again, the barrier is encouraged to recede. This is repeated several times.

Actual techniques will not be described here, but those interested can find them in several authors[1, 2, 3].

Isometric Contraction (Muscle Energy) Techniques

These will be described as an alternative to high velocity treatment. The principle is that the joint is taken up to the barrier in all three planes; the patient is then instructed to attempt to push in the opposite direction away from the barrier. The physician resists this movement with an equal and opposite counterforce. The amount of force varies with the size of the muscle concerned but need never be more than moderate. The manoeuvre ought to be painless. After a short period of resisted contraction, the patient is instructed to relax and the counterforce is stopped at the same moment. At no time must the physician push the joint through the barrier.

When full relaxation has occurred, the physician takes the joint to the new barrier. In most patients there are two phases of relaxation. At first they merely stop pushing and, before she will do so, it is often necessary to ask the patient to relax fully. When the new barrier is found and lightly engaged, the process is repeated and may be done three, four or sometimes more times, if progress is being made. A very similar technique can be used to obtain relaxation in tight muscles, for instance, the hamstrings, or the adductor muscles of the thigh. Isometric exercises of this kind away from the barrier are much the best form of exercise for the "frozen shoulder".

Hamstring stretching by this method can be used when the forward flexion test for the sacro-iliac joint is vitiated by unilateral tightness. This is done as follows: (Fig. 41)

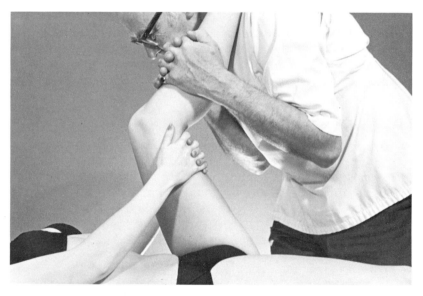

Fig. 41 Isometric technique for stretching left hamstring muscles.

1 The patient lies supine.
2 You stand on the same side as the bad leg, facing the head of the table.
3 You flex the hip and knee on the bad side until she can clasp her hands behind the back of the thigh, to maintain the flexion of the hip.
4 You then extend the knee to the barrier and, with as much crouch as is necessary, rest the calf on your near shoulder.
5 Tell the patient to press down on your shoulder, by contracting her hamstrings.

6 After a few seconds you tell her to relax.
7 After full relaxation you raise your shoulder to the new barrier.
8 Repeat three or four times.

It will often be found that sufficient stretching has been obtained so that the forward flexion test can be performed more accurately.

The reason for the success of isometric contraction is probably that in some way it resets the "gain" in the gamma system which controls the length of the muscle fibres. The spindle is "cheated" into thinking that the muscle has shortened during the contraction and, on relaxation, allows some lengthening. It is most important that the counterforce should be equal to the patient effort and, therefore, unyielding. Failure to maintain the position, and failure to reach the barrier accurately, will make the treatment less effective. It may be necessary to caution the patient not to use too much force.

If the anatomy of any muscle is known, it is possible to devise an isometric technique to stretch it.

Difficulties

Often the first problem met by the orthodox physician when he encounters manipulation is the concept that it is possible to treat a single spinal joint on its own merits (or for its own faults!). The techniques of examination and treatment are very largely concerned with methods, first of making a specific diagnosis; secondly, of applying a specific treatment.

Methods which enable one to make a diagnosis have been described and others could be added. Methods of treatment will be described in the next chapters.

Localisation of Force

A cabinet maker does not drive home a nail all the way with the simple hammer, if he did he would mark the wood around the nail with the final blows. He uses a nail punch to finish the job so that there is only a small hole to fill instead of the mark of the face of the hammer.

In the same way a manipulator localises the force to the joint that is to be moved, otherwise neighbouring structures might be harmed. One of the reasons for the scant success of traction is that it cannot be accurately localised. It wastes most, and often all, of its effect on neighbouring mobile joints and may have little or no effect on the one causing the trouble. Marked separation can be seen at normal joints if x-rays are taken while the patient is on traction.

Force is localised by positioning the patient. The third law tells us that motion of a spinal joint in any plane will limit the range of motion in the other planes. This can be applied in such a way that on either side of the lesion, movement of the joints is prevented in the direction of the intended force. This procedure is known as locking and the concept involved is helpful when one is considering high velocity manipulation. The concept of joint locking is not the same as that of the barrier described in Chapter 3. Locking is what one can do to a normal joint. The pathological barrier is what one finds in an abnormal joint. Locking of course, involves taking the normal joint up to one part of its physiological barrier- possibly even to the anatomical barrier.

Locking can be produced by taking movement in any plane as far as it will go, e.g. flexion. The division of a movement into three planes at right angles to each other is a descriptive device which nature does not recognize. Locking can be produced in side bending—rotation, with or without flexion or extension, providing the movement at that joint is taken to its limit in the particular direction.

Here, however, is a difficulty. Spinal joints do not move separately, they are like traffic lights that are linked together. Long before the first joint reaches the limit of its movement, the next one has started to move. It is easy to go too far and at least partially lock the joint that one is trying to move. One of the things one learns by experience is how far to go. In order to decide how far to go one must monitor with one's fingers. Monitoring can be by either or both of two changes. First the movement of the joint. Secondly the tissue tension around the joint. Accuracy in this kind of palpation is much improved by practice.

All movements must be made by the manipulator with the patient relaxed. Any attempt to help on the part of the patient will make it impossible for the manipulator to feel accurately.

For a start it is useful to use the following method:

When positioning the patient, by whatever movement is appropriate, the movement is continued until the tissue tension at the problem joint is felt to increase. Alternatively one can say until the problem joint ought to move, judging by the movement of the ones below and above. At that point one reverses the movement slightly so that the tissue tension at the *next* level begins to relax or the movement at the *next* level is partly undone. By next level is meant the next joint in the direction from which locking is being produced, e.g. if one is locking up to L2–3 from below (in order to manipulate the L2–3 joint), the tension and movement should be partly taken out from the L3–4 joint. The commonest mistake among beginners is to go too far and make their task more difficult by locking the problem joint!

Application of Force

Nature has equipped the vertebrae with a number of small levers by which they can be moved. The most useful are the spinous and transverse processes in the lumbar and thoracic regions and the articular pillars (articular or lateral masses) in the neck.

The total range of movement at a single spinal joint is variable but always small. (See Ch. 2 for figures). To overcome the stiffness and make the joint move may require some force. In order to avoid damage the force must be stopped as soon as the movement has happened. With a short lever this is difficult. The principle of the lever is that if one doubles its length, one halves the force required at its distal end and doubles the range through which that end should be moved.

It is obvious therefore, that a longer lever would have great advantages, the force required would be less and the distance travelled greater, making control of the force much easier. By accurate locking from above down and from below up to the problem joint one can construct such a long lever and apply one's force at a distance, monitoring with the fingers over the joint itself.

Flexion is the movement most commonly used to lock the spine up to the lesion in the lumbar region. Theoretically it would be possible to use flexion from above also. A moment's thought, however, will show that, because we are dealing with a living subject, a slight movement on the part of the patient could easily cause the problem joint to be flexed also. A different position, usually sidebending-rotation, is therefore used.

There are techniques of applying high velocity thrust directly to the transverse or spinous processes (or to the articular pillars in the neck). These can be called short lever techniques. When one uses such a thrust it is most important that the amplitude (distance travelled by the force) should be very strictly controlled. Some hybrid techniques will also be described where a long lever is used on one side of the joint and a short lever on the other. If possible the force is applied to the long lever side, as this gives the advantage of easier control.

Caution

A careful re-examination is essential before each treatment. A successful treatment will alter the situation although the same joint may need further attention.

When a patient is in acute pain, the abnormal muscle tension may be widespread and it is easy to be mistaken as to the precise level of the main problem. In such circumstances it may well be that the subsequent examinations will show that the most important level is not quite where it originally appeared to be.

Even when the correct joint was treated initially it is common to find that, on subsequent examinations, other joints needing treatment are found. If there is an old somatic dysfunction at one level, it may happen that a fresh injury will cause dysfunction at another joint. Very often it will be found that it will be necessary to find and treat the old joint before the new one will stay better. This happens even when the two joints are widely separated. It is the main reason for seeking and treating loss of function rather than "chasing the pain".

Retesting

It is good practice always to re-examine the part after any manipulation. If there is no change some other procedure or a repeat treatment may be helpful.

REFERENCES

1 Stoddard, A. (1959), *Manual of Osteopathic Technique*, London, Hutchinson.
2 Maitland, G. D. (1964), *Vertebral Manipulation*, London, Butterworth.
3 Maigne, R. (1972), *Orthopedic Medicine* Springfield, Ill., Thomas.

6

Treatment of the Joints of the Pelvis

Nomenclature

A variety of terms are used to describe the different types of dysfunction of joints in the pelvic ring. For the sake of simplicity the author will follow the orthodox medical profession. The term sacro-iliac will be used to include those sometimes known as ilio-sacral. The terms anterior and posterior innominate will be used where some might prefer posterior and anterior sacrum and some other names.

Priorities

The symphysis pubis is a hinge on the proper function of which depends much of pelvic function. Partly for this reason disturbances of this joint are treated first. The position of the sacrum between the ilia is treated next and if there then remains any positional abnormality in the innominates, these are treated last.

Because disturbances of function in the pelvis must affect the lumbar joints, and therefore the whole spine, it is usually considered wise to deal with the pelvic dysfunction first. This is true even if there are no symptoms in the lower back or hip region.

For many years the author used a much simplified approach. The sacro-iliac joints were treated by mobilising the ilium on the sacrum in one or other direction. Diagnosis was made by finding sacro-iliac joint stiffness, and often tenderness, and a a failure of the expected response to lumbar treatment.

There appears to be no doubt that many of the described pelvic dysfunctions will respond to a combination of such sacro-iliac and lumbar treatment. The more specific treatment of the pelvic joints is necessary for those who do not respond and probably gives more rapid results even in those that would respond.

Diagnosis

This has been described in Chapter 3. The diagnosis of dysfunction in the pelvis depends on the findings of positional abnormalities and loss of movement.

A positive forward flexion test suggests stiffness in the sacroiliac joint but is not necessarily found in those with dysfunction at the symphysis. Up and down motion of one pubic bone on the other can be tested by gripping the medial end of the superior ramus between forefinger and thumb on each side and attempting to move one bone on the other. The range of movement is very small.

The diagnosis of symphysis dysfunction is usually made by finding an abnormality of position. The forward flexion test when positive, indicates which is the side needing treatment.

If the pubic bones are level or if, after they have been treated and corrected, the forward flexion test is again positive, the patient is turned to the prone position and the relations of the sacrum to the ilia are examined. It will sometimes be found that the forward flexion test is now positive on the other side.

The main diagnostic points are:

1 The depth of the sulcus (medial to the posterior superior spine).
2 The position of the inferior lateral angle of the sacrum on each side. Is one more posterior or more inferior than the other?
3 The relative length of the legs at the medial malleolus.
4 The depth of the lumbar lordosis and whether the lumbar spine springs easily.

Additional help may be obtained from the backward bending test and the relative positions of the posterior superior spines— both up and down and front to back.

If the ILA position is the same on the two sides, or, if after this has been dealt with and the repeated forward flexion test is still positive, the patient is turned supine. The height (with reference to the anatomical position) of the anterior superior iliac spines may indicate the presence of an innominate dysfunction.

It is found clinically that a posterior innominate is much more common on the left than on the right. Forward torsion of the sacrum on the left oblique axis is common. Other torsions are relatively uncommon. In this connection the author's observation is of interest that a short right leg is twice as common as a short left leg in over 1000 patients complaining of back pain.

Treatment

1 Elevated pubis on the left—Isometric technique (Fig. 42)

Diagnostic points:
1 *Standing* flexion test positive on the left.
2 *Supine* pubic tubercle higher on the left.

Technique:
1 Patient lies supine on the left side of the table with her left leg hanging over the side.
2 You stand to her left facing her head and support her left leg by gripping it lightly, just above the ankle, between your legs.
3 With your left hand stabilise her right ASIS.
4 With your right hand "take up the slack" by pressing her left knee down to the barrier (as far as it will easily go). Hold it there.
5 Tell her to attempt to raise her left leg straight and resist with an equal, opposite force. Hold for a few seconds.
6 When she relaxes fully you take up the slack by pressing down on the knee.
7 Repeat steps 5 and 6 twice or three times.

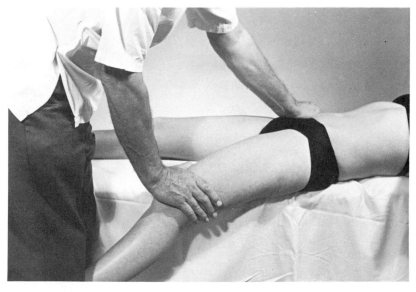

Fig. 42 Treatment of elevated left pubis.

NOTE:

(1) Wait for full relaxation. There are often two phases, first she stops pushing and secondly she really relaxes. The patient may need to be told a second time to relax fully.

(2) When she relaxes let go your counterforce but maintain the position of the knee.

(3) When you take up the slack the object is to go up to *not* through the barrier and it is important to be gentle.

(4) An elevated pubis is always accompanied by a dysfunction in the sacro-iliac joint, usually (but not always) a posterior innominate on the same side.

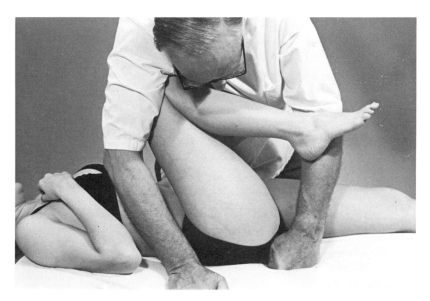

Fig. 43 Treatment of right depressed pubis.

2 Depressed pubis on the right—Isometric technique (Fig. 43)
Diagnostic points:

1 *Standing* flexion test positive on the right.

2 *Supine* pubic tubercle lower on the right (or higher on the left).

Technique:

1 Patient lies supine with right knee and hip fully flexed.

2 You stand to her left and place her knee in your right axilla holding the right side of the table with your right hand.

3 Place your left fist against her right ischial tuberosity and press craniad.
4 Instruct her to try to push you away with her knee.
5 After a few seconds both relax but you hold the position.
6 When she relaxes fully you take up the slack by flexing the hip.
7 Repeat steps 4, 5 and 6 twice or three times.

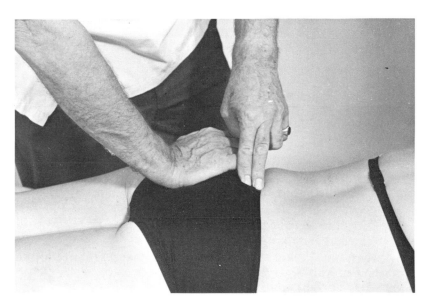

Fig. 44 Treatment of unilateral sacral flexion on the left.

3 Unilateral sacral flexion on the left (Fig. 44)
Diagnostic points:
1 *Sitting* forward flexion test usually positive on the left.
2 *Prone*
   (a) left inferior lateral angle of sacrum (ILA) relatively inferior and slightly posterior,
   (b) left sulcus deep,
   (c) left medial malleolus inferior (caudad)
Technique:
1 Patient lies prone.
2 You stand to her left and monitor left sacro-iliac movement with your left hand—fingers in sulcus.
3 With your right hand adjust the position of her left leg to give maximum feeling of freedom in SI joint. This requires

some abduction and internal rotation at the hip, monitored by the fingers of your left hand.

4 With the heel of your right hand press down on her left ILA in the direction that appears to give maximum movement under your left fingers. Your right elbow should be straight.

5 Have the patient take a deep breath and hold it. Maintain the pressure.

6 Have her breathe out slowly while you maintain the pressure.

7 Repeat steps 5 and 6 three times.

4 Forward sacral torsion on the left axis (left on left) (Fig. 45)
Diagnostic points:

1 *Sitting* flexion test usually positive on left.

2 *Prone*

   (a) left ILA relatively posterior and slightly inferior,

   (b) left sulcus shallow,

   (c) lumbar lordosis increased and negative backward bending test,

   (d) left medial malleolus superior (craniad).

Technique:

1 Patient lies prone close to the table edge on her right with her right arm hanging over the side.

2 You stand facing her right side and lift her right hip enough to bend up both legs so that hips and knees are flexed to about a right angle.

3 You support and control her knees with your thigh, hip or abdomen.

4 You flex her legs together until movement is felt at the lumbosacral junction with your left hand.

5 Tell the patient to take a deep breath and as she lets it out, to reach for the floor with her right hand. This you assist by pressure downwards with your right hand on the back of her right shoulder.

6 Repeat the breathing movement twice and hold the rotation.

7 With your left hand move her feet together off the table and depress them to produce a left side bend in the lumbar spine and at the lumbosacral junction.

8 Have her attempt to raise her feet toward the ceiling against your resistance and relax.

9 As she relaxes you take up the slack.

10 Repeat steps 8 and 9 twice or three times.

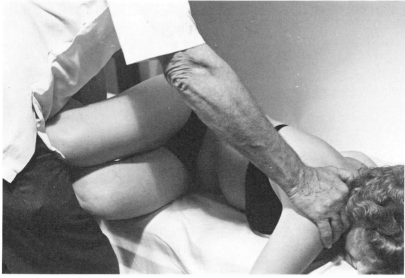

(a)

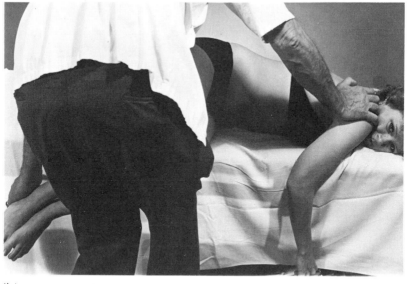

(b)

Fig. 45 Treatment of forward sacral torsion on the left axis (left on left torsion.) (a) Shows initial position during effort to obtain full left rotation of the trunk. (b) Shows position for isometric effort to produce left sidebending. Note the position of the patient's feet and the operator's hand used to resist the effort.

NOTE:

In the first manoeuvre the spinal column is brought into the same rotation as the sacrum. When the sacrum and lumbar spine are "lined up" in neutral flexion-extension, the addition of left sidebending forces the sacrum to rotate to the right according to the first law of spinal motion.

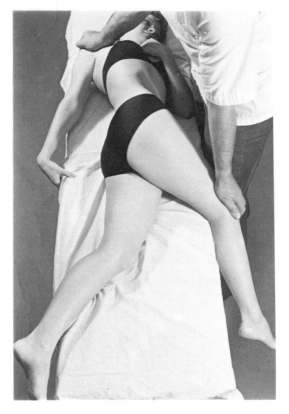

Fig. 46 Treatment of backward sacral torsion on the left axis (right on left torsion). Note the extension of the left hip and spine and the full right rotation of the trunk.

5 Backward sacral torsion on the left axis (right on left) (Fig. 46)
Diagnostic points:
1 *Sitting* flexion test may be positive on either side.
2 *Prone*
   (a) right ILA posterior and slightly inferior,
   (b) right sulcus shallow,
   (c) lumbar lordosis flat and backward bending test positive,
   (d) right medial malleolus superior (craniad).

NOTE:

The only difference between right on left (backward) and right on right torsion (forward) is in the state of the lordosis and in the confirmatory backward bending test.

Technique:
1 Patient lies on her left side close to the front of the table.
2 You stand facing her and pull her left arm forward so that her left shoulder is in front of her trunk.
3 Extend her left leg fully and allow her right leg to lie in front of it.
4 Monitor the lumbosacral joint with your right hand while you hyperextend her left hip until lumbosacral motion is felt.
5 Move your right hand to the front of her right shoulder and have her breathe out as you rotate her shoulders to the right as far as possible. Repeat once or twice.
6 Have her grasp the back edge of the table with her right hand.
7 With your left hand drop her right leg off the front of the table and depress her knee as far as it will go.
8 Have her attempt to raise her right knee against your unyielding resistance and then relax.
9 On full relaxation you take up the slack.
10 Repeat steps 8 and 9 three or four times.

NOTE:

The principles of correction her are the same as for the forward torsion. The lumbar spine is first "lined up" with the sacrum and the correction made by sidebending.

6 Left posterior innominate
Diagnostic points:
1 *Standing* flexion test positive on the left.
2 *Prone*
(a) ILA symmetrical,
(b) left sulcus deep,
(c) left PSIS relatively inferior and posterior.
3 *Supine*
(a) left ASIS relatively superior and posterior,
(b) left medial malleolus superior (craniad).
Technique:
(A) Isometric (with high velocity variant) (Fig. 47)

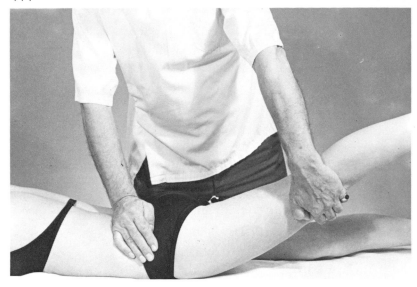

Fig. 47 Prone technique for treatment of a left posterior innominate.

1 Patient lies prone.
2 You stand on her right.
3 With your left hand lift her left leg at the knee and abduct at the hip to the point of maximum freedom in the left sacro-iliac joint (monitored by the right fingers).
4 With your right hand steady her left iliac crest in front of the posterior spine.
5 With your left hand lift her left leg to the barrier and at the same time press down (anteriorly) on the iliac crest with your right hand.
6 Have the patient attempt to pull her leg down to the table while you prevent movement by an equal and opposite force.
6a Alternative high velocity variation—At the end of exhalation you make a simultaneous high velocity, low amplitude thrust downwards with your right hand on the iliac crest and upwards with your left hand under the left knee. (Omit steps 7 and 8).
7 Have her relax but do not lose the position. When she relaxes take up the slack by elevating her left leg as far as it will go without moving the sacrum (i.e. to the new barrier).
8 Repeat steps 6 and 7 two or three times.

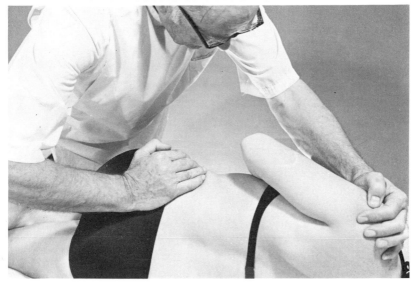

Fig. 48 Side lying technique for treatment of a left posterior innominate.

(B) High Velocity (Fig. 48)

    1 The patient lies on her right side.

    2 You stand in front of her.

    3 With your left hand pull her left shoulder forwards.

    4 With your right hand bend up her left knee and hip so that the left foot rests in her right popliteal fossa, and the left knee drops over the edge of the table.

    5 Place your left hand on the front of her left shoulder and ease the trunk into full left rotation in order to lock the spine down to the lumbosacral joint.

    6 With your right pisiform make contact with the lower part of her left posterior iliac spine with the forearm pointing backwards at an angle of about thirty degrees to the long axis of the body and horizontal.

    7 The thrust is given by a high velocity, low amplitude movement of the right forearm and hand thrusting craniad and forwards on the lower part of the posterior iliac spine while the left hand slightly increases the rotation of the trunk.

NOTE:

    In resistant cases a gapping of the sacro-iliac joint can be produced by you pressing downward with your left knee on her left knee, increasing the adduction of the hip.

7 Left anterior innominate

Diagnostic points:
1 *Standing* flexion test positive on the left.
2 *Prone*
   (a) ILA symmetrical,
   (b) left sulcus shallow,
   (c) left PSIS relatively anterior and superior.
3 *Supine*
   (a) left ASIS relatively inferior and anterior,
   (b) left medial malleolus inferior (caudad).

Technique:
(A) Isometric (Fig. 49)
   1 Patient lies on her right side.
   2 You stand facing her.
   3 With your left hand bend up her left knee and hip to the limit and control with your abdomen or thigh.
   4 With your right hand monitor movement at her left sacro-iliac joint.
   5 Instruct the patient to try to straighten her leg, resist the movement.
   6 Both relax and take up the slack by increasing hip flexion.
   7 Repeat steps 5 and 6 two or three times.

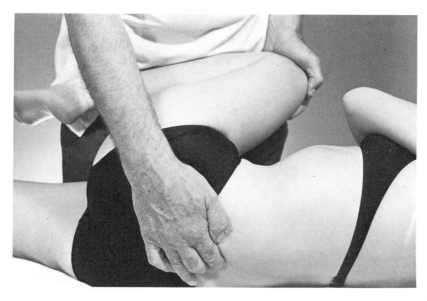

Fig. 49 Isometric treatment for a left anterior innominate.

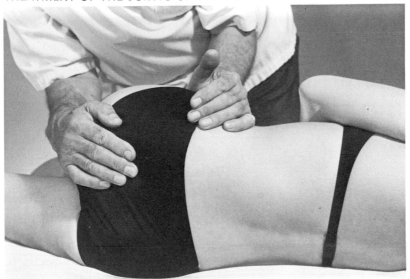

Fig. 50 Thrusting treatment for a left anterior innominate.

(B) High Velocity (Fig. 50)
   1 Patient lies on her right side.
   2 You stand facing her.
   3 Position her right leg straight on the table.
   4 Bend her left hip so that the leg hangs over the table edge.
   5 With your right hand grasp her left ischial tuberosity and
      with your left hand press backwards on the anterior part
      of her left iliac crest.
   6 Increase tension by pulling forward with your right hand.
      When the barrier is engaged give a high velocity low
      amplitude thrust forwards with the right hand.

7

Treatment of the Lumbar Spine

Locking of neighbouring joints is important and more so as one goes higher up the spine. When the author started he found it difficult to get above T11–12 but with experience the second technique can be used for two or three joints higher.

The first technique is hybrid and only requires accurate locking on the long lever side. Correct positioning, however, will much assist the movement. It requires a more awkward position for the manipulator and the author no longer uses it except in demonstration.

Both techniques use rotation as the main corrective force and it must be remembered that there is only a very small range of rotation at any of the lumbar joints. The techniques are essentially similar but the point of application of the caudad force is different.

In patients who have severe pain and who cannot relax, manipulation can sometimes be made possible by a small caudal epidural injection of local anaesthetic. It is possible to invent a set of circumstances that would justify a general anaesthetic. In practice it is "never" necessary. General anaesthetic has the disadvantage that it may produce enough relaxation to make locking more difficult. It can also remove protective muscle spasm over possibly unsuspected destructive bone lesions.

Acute cases should not be subjected to high velocity manipulation except by those with experience.

1 *Simplified treatment using diagnosis by motion loss and muscle tension.*

(A) Hybrid technique: (Figs. 51, 52)

This will be described for a problem at the L3–4 joint with the maximal tension on the right side.

 1 The patient lies on her left side.

 2 You stand facing her.

3 With your left hand flex her right hip and knee. Control the degree of flexion and support the knee either with your abdomen or with your left hand.

4 With your right hand palpate the interspinous ligament between L3 and 4.

5 Flex her right hip until movement begins at the L3-4 joint and then remove that movement by extending the hip slightly. Ensure that the patient is relaxed during this positioning.

6 Without losing the flexion put down her right leg so that it hangs freely over the side of the table. If she seems likely to move it, lock it in position by putting one leg on each side of it.

7 Move your left hand to palpate the L2-3 interspinous ligament.

8 With your right hand grasp her under (left) arm, pull her shoulder forward and continue until movement is felt at the L2-3 level (one level up from the joint to be treated). Again the patient must be relaxed. This is the long lever.

The spine is now locked from below by flexion and from above by rotation-sidebending.

9 Place your left hand with the wrist extended so that the pisiform bone contacts the right transverse process of her 4th lumbar vertebra. The forearm should be horizontal and perpendicular to the length of the body.

10 With your right hand on the front of her right shoulder press backward to take up the slack.

11 Have the patient breath deeply in and out three times. Each time you take up more slack as she relaxes.

12 Perform the correction with a short sharp thrust anteriorly (towards you) with your left pisiform on the transverse process of L4. The counter thrust is by your right hand on the front of her right shoulder exaggerating the position. Thrust and counterthrust must be simultaneous.

(B) Long lever technique: (Fig. 53)

This will be described for the same problem (L3-4 joint) with maximal tension on the right side.

Steps 1 to 8 as in (A). Accurate performance of steps 3, 4 and 5 is now more important.

9 With the fingers of the left hand palpating the L3-4

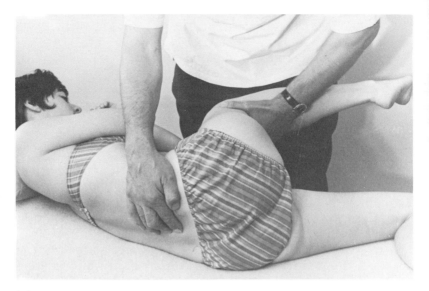

(a)

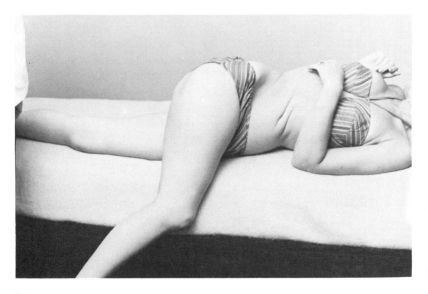

(b)

Fig. 51 Locking in the lumbar spine. (a) Lumbar locking from below.
(b) After lumbar locking from below. (c) Locking from above down to the
lumbar region.

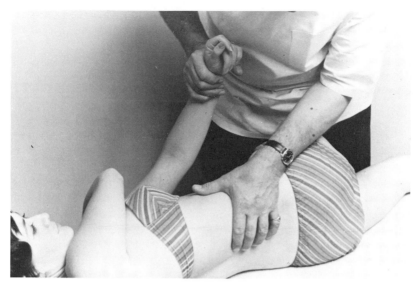

(c)

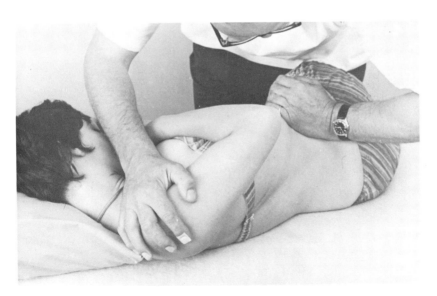

Fig. 52 Position for thrusting in the hybrid technique.

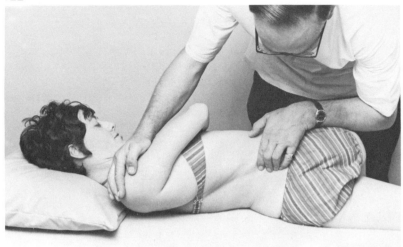

(a)

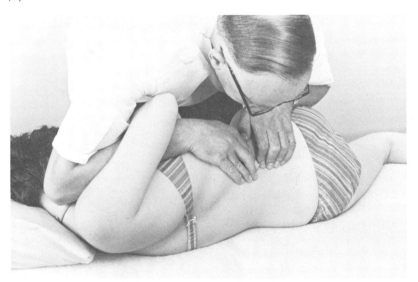

(b)

Fig. 53 Position for thrusting in the long lever technique. (a) Using the hand on the shoulder. (b) Using the elbow on the shoulder.

level rest the back of your left forearm on her right buttock so that with it pressure can be exerted at a point roughly midway between her anterior superior iliac spine and her ischial tuberosity.

10a With your right hand on the front of her right shoulder press backward to take up the slack.

10b Put your right arm through her right axilla so that your fingers can palpate the spinous process of L3 while your elbow is in position to press on the front of her right shoulder to take up the slack.

11 Have the patient breathe deeply in and out three times. Each time you take up more slack as she relaxes.

12 Perform the correction by a thrust with the body weight downwards on the patient producing simultaneous forward rotation of her pelvis (and locked lower lumbar joints) and backward rotation of her shoulder and upper spine.

NOTE:

(1) For the lumbo-sacral joint the second technique may always be used because no inferior locking is appropriate.

(2) For the L4–5 level care must be taken with step 4 or the joint may inadvertently be locked.

(3) The importance of the patient's relaxation cannot be over-emphasised. This, indeed, is the main reason for the inclusion of step 11. If she attempts to hold up the dependent leg, the manipulation will fail unless a force is used that is greater than advisable.

2 *Specific treatment using results of positional diagnosis.* (See p. 67)

There are three possible positions:

1 Side bending-rotation in neutral. Rotation will be to the convexity of the side bend (Law I).

2 Side bending-rotation in hyperflexion. Rotation will be to the concavity (Law II).

3 Side bending-rotation in extension. Rotation will be to the concavity (Law II).

The principle in high velocity treatment is to take the problem joint up to the barrier and then to use a thrust to move through where the barrier was. The principle in isometric treatment is to take the joint up to the barrier and then to make the barrier recede by using resisted muscle effort. The latter is more complex because the barrier must be engaged in all three planes. The effectiveness of isometric treatment depends largely on the accuracy of engagement of the barrier. In this connection it should be pointed out that the position of the barrier in the anteroposterior (flexion-extension or sagittal) plane will not be the same if the amount of side bending or rotation is changed.

The easiest way to perform a "lumbar roll" as in the first two techniques is to rotate the pelvis forward and the shoulders back. This produces a rotation of the trunk away from the side on which the patient is lying.

If, as in the first two techniques, the under shoulder is pulled forwards, there is a small side bend towards the table. This side bend is then in the opposite direction to the rotation produced by a lumbar roll manipulation. This is the proper sense for the treatment of neutral problems. In order to treat extension or flexion problems the reverse is needed and the patient therefore lies with the shoulder directly under her and the head supported on her arm or on a pillow. Suppose she has a flexion lesion of L3–4 sidebent and rotated to the right, in order to reach the side bending-rotation barrier the patient must lie on her right side. This encourages side bending to the left so long as the right shoulder is not pulled out from under her. When the lumbar roll rotation is applied, she is also rotated to the left. Because of the direction of rotation required, neutral lesions are also treated with the patient lying on the involved side.

(C) Lumber roll technique: for treatment of the lumbar spine in "neutral": (Type I lesion)

Described for a right rotated L3.

(Restriction of rotation to the left.) (Fig. 54)

Diagnostic points:

1 Several rotated vertebrae.

2 No exaggeration of position on flexion or extension.

High velocity method:

1 The patient lies on her right side.

2 You stand facing her.

3 With your right hand monitor for movement at the L3–4 interspinous ligament (ISL).

4 With your left hand take hold of her right arm at the elbow and pull it towards you until movement is felt with the fingers of the right hand at L3–4.

5 Thread your left arm through her left axilla and rest your forearm against the front of her left shoulder.

6 With your right hand bend her left hip until her foot lies behind her right knee.

7 Move your right forearm so that it rests on her left buttock halfway between the ASIS and the ischial tuberosity. Both hands can now be used to monitor the L3–4 interspace.

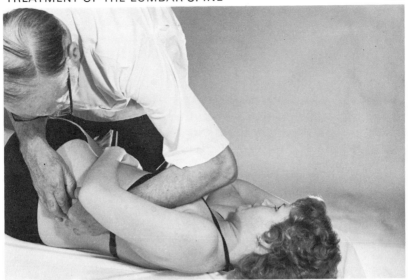

Fig. 54 Lumbar roll technique for L3 rotated to the right in neutral flexion. Note that the right shoulder has been "pulled out from under her".

    8 Have the patient breathe deeply in and out three times. Each time take up the slack as she relaxes by easing her left hip forwards and her right hip back.

    9 Apply a short, sharp thrust equally with your left forearm backwards on the shoulder and your right forearm forwards on the buttock.

Mitchell[1], advises that this should be done by "dropping your weight equally through both arms, straight down on the patient."

Isometric method:

    Steps 1 to 8 as in high velocity treatment.

    9 Have the patient grip the back edge of the table with her left hand and instruct her to push her left knee upwards (abduct the thigh) against your unyielding resistance.

    10 Both relax but do not lose the position. Take up the rotatory slack.

    11 Repeat steps 9 and 10 twice or three times.

(D) Lumbar roll technique for treatment of a lumbar spine with restricted flexion: (Type II lesion)

    Described for a right rotated L3 (restriction of rotation and sidebending to the left). (Fig. 55)

Diagnostic points:

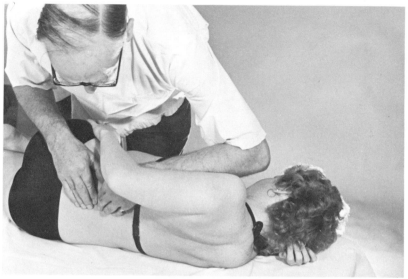

Fig. 55 Lumbar roll technique for L3 rotated to the right with restricted flexion. Note that she is lying on her right shoulder.

1 A single rotated vertebra.
2 The deformity is exaggerated by flexion of the spine.
High velocity method:
    1 The patient lies on her right side with her head supported on a pillow or on her arm.
    2 You stand facing her. Do not pull her left shoulder forward.
    3 Thread your left arm through her left axilla and with your left hand monitor movement at the L3–4 interspace.
    4 With your right hand flex her left leg until her foot rests behind her right knee.
    5 Move your right hand to flex her right hip until movement begins to be felt with your left hand.
    6 Move your right forearm so that it rests on her left buttock midway between the ASIS and the ischial tuberosity.
    7 Have the patient breathe deeply in and out three times. Each time as she relaxes take up the slack.
    8 Apply a short, sharp thrust equally with your left forearm backward on the shoulder and your right forearm forward on the buttock.
Isometric method:
    Steps 1 to 7 as in high velocity treatment.
      8 Have the patient grip the back edge of the table with

her left hand and push her left knee upwards (abduct
the thigh) against your unyielding resistance.
9 Both relax, but do not lose the position. Take up the
rotatory slack.
10 Repeat steps 8 and 9 twice or three times.

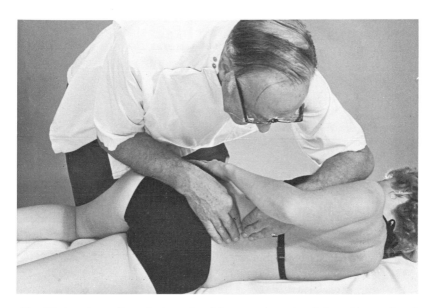

Fig. 56 Lumbar roll technique for L3 rotated to the right with restricted
extension. Note the extended right hip and leg.

(E) Lumbar roll technique for treatment of a lumbar spine
with restricted extension: (Type II)
Described for a right rotated L3. (Fig. 56)
Diagnostic points:
1 A single rotated vertebra.
2 The deformity is exaggerated by extension of the spine.
High velocity method:
1 The patient lies on her right side near the front edge of the
table and with her head supported on a pillow or on her
arm.
2 You stand facing her. Do not pull her left shoulder
forward.
3 Thread your left arm through her left axilla and with
your left hand monitor movement at the L3–4 interspace.
4 With your right hand flex her left leg until her foot rests
in front of her right knee.

5 With your right hand push her right leg backwards so that the spine is extended until movement is felt with the left hand. She must be relaxed during this movement.

6 Move your right forearm so that it rests on her left buttock, midway between the ASIS and the ischial tuberosity.

7 Have the patient breathe deeply in and out three times. Each time as she relaxes take up the slack.

8 Apply a short sharp thrust equally with your left forearm backward on the shoulder and your right forearm forwards on the buttock.

Isometric method:

Steps 1 to 7 as in high velocity treatment.

8 Have the patient grip the back edge of the table with her left hand and push her right knee upwards (abduct the thigh) against your unyielding resistance.

9 Both relax, but do not lose the position. When she relaxes fully, take up the rotatory slack.

10 Repeat steps 8 and 9 twice or three times.

(F) Sitting technique for treatment of lumbar spine in neutral: (Type I lesion)

Described for a right rotated L3. (Fig. 57)

For diagnostic points see (C) above.

High velocity method:

1 The patient sits astride the end of the table.

2 You stand behind her with a wide stance adjusted so that you can support your right elbow with your right hip.

3 You control her trunk movement with your left arm. Reach through her left axilla and across her front to grasp her right shoulder. She should grasp her own left shoulder with her right hand.

4 Contact the right transverse process of L3 with the base of your right thenar eminence.

5 With the lumbar spine in neutral (slight flexion) bring her into left rotation and right sidebending until you feel the tension accumulate under your right thenar eminence. Keep her weight over her hips as far as possible.

6 The thrust is given by a simultaneous movement increasing left rotation and right sidebending and a forward push with your right hand on the transverse process of L3.

Isometric method:

Steps 1 to 5 as in the high velocity method.

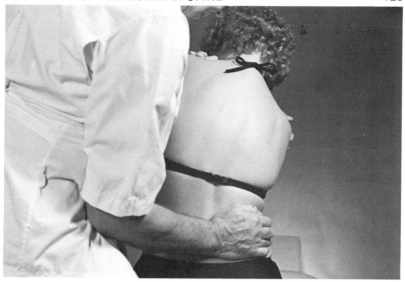

Fig. 57 Sitting technique for L3 rotated to the right in neutral flexion. Note the position of left rotation and *right* sidebending.

6 Have the patient attempt to straighten the sidebending or rotation or both while you resist.

7 After a few seconds have her relax and stop your counterforce without losing the position.

8 When she has relaxed fully you take up the slack in sidebending and rotation.

9 Repeat steps 7 and 8 two or three times.

10 Finally have her bend forward to touch the table top with her right shoulder.

NOTE:

(1) Compare thoracic techniques which are very similar.

(2) A stool may be used in which case the patient's feet must be firmly on the floor and the end point of step 10 is to have her touch the floor with her right hand.

(G) Sitting technique for a lumbar spine with restricted flexion: (Type II lesion)

Described for a right rotated L3. (Fig. 58)

For diagnostic points see (D) above.

1 The patient sits on a stool or chair, feet on the floor and legs apart. The knees should be at about a right angle. She should be slightly slumped forward, arms hanging, the right between her legs, the left by her side.

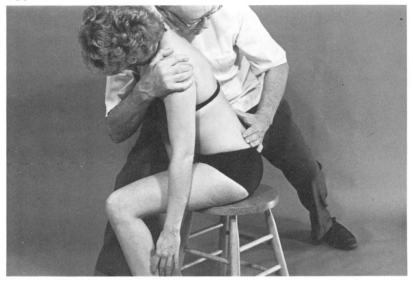

Fig. 58 Sitting technique for L3 rotated to the right with restricted flexion. This is the position at the end of step 7.

2 You stand facing her right side, put your right foot between her feet.

3 Lean a little forward to grasp her left shoulder with your right hand and press your right shoulder against her right shoulder.

4 Use your left hand to monitor movement at the L3–4 joint.

5 So adjust her slump position that L3 becomes the vertebra most prominent posteriorly.

6 Maintain the flexion and sidebend her to the left, away from you. To maintain your balance you will need to pull some of her weight over her right hip.

7 Maintain the flexion and sidebending. Add rotation to the left until motion is felt by your left hand.

8 Have her attempt to reach for the floor with her left hand while you resist.

9 After a few seconds have her relax. Then take up the slack in sidebending, then rotation then flexion.

10 Repeat steps 8 and 9 two or three times.

11 Have her push against you with her right shoulder while you resist.

12 After a few seconds have her relax. Then take up the slack as before.

13 Repeat steps 11 and 12 two or three times.

14 Maintain her position. Move your right foot out so that you are standing beside her. Move your right hand to the front of her right shoulder and your left hand to the back of her left shoulder.

15 Flex her, maintaining the rotation, by having her reach for the floor with her right hand. Then bring down the left shoulder by having her reach for the floor with her left hand.

16 Finally return her to the seated erect position passively against her slight resistance.

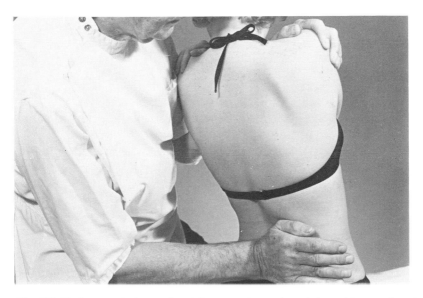

Fig. 59 Sitting technique for L3 rotated to the right with restricted extension.

(H) Sitting technique for lumbar spine with restricted extension (in hyperflexion). (Type II lesion)

Described for a right rotated L3. (Fig. 59)

For diagnostic points see (E) above.

High velocity method:

1 The patient sits astride the end of the table.

2 You stand behind her with a wide stance adjusted so that you can support your right elbow with your right hip.

3 You control her trunk movement with your left arm.

Reach through her left axilla and across her front to grasp her right shoulder. She should grasp her left shoulder with her right hand.

4 Contact the left side of the spinous process or the right transverse process of L3 with the base of your right thenar eminence.

5 Bring her into left rotation and left sidebending and extension until the tension accumulates under your right thenar eminence. Keep her weight over her hips as much as possible.

6 Thrust simultaneously with your right hand (supported by the hip) and by increasing the sidebending, rotation and extension of her trunk.

NOTE:

The backward bending required is often best achieved by having her arch her back.

Isometric method:

Steps 1 to 5 as in high velocity method.

- 6 Have the patient attempt to straighten her position against your unyielding resistance.

7 After a few seconds have her relax and stop your counter-force without losing the position.

8 When she has relaxed fully, you take up the slack in all three planes.

9 Repeat steps 7 and 8 two or three times.

NOTE:

It is often better to attempt to straighten the sidebending and rotation first and to deal with the sagittal plane movement afterwards.

REFERENCE

Mitchell, F. L., Moran, P. S. and Pruzzo, M. T. (1973), *An evaluation and treatment manual of osteopathic manupulative procedure*, 2nd Ed. Institute for continuing education in Osteopathic Principles, Kansas City, Missouri.

8

Treatment of the Thoracic Spine

The thoracic spine is complicated by the presence of the ribs and the costo-vertebral joints. Overall movement is much restricted by the rib cage. What is more, the intercostal and costo-vertebral muscles can be affected by persistent tightness in the same way as the muscles of the spine itself.

Tightness in the intercostal muscles with restriction of rib motion can cause symptoms that closely resemble those produced by similar tension in the corresponding spinal muscles. Often the two go together, indeed it is rare to find a stiff rib joint without a similar problem in the intervertebral joint. The reverse is not true, however, intervertebral joints in the thoracic spine often give trouble without any rib involvement.

The thoracic spine should be considered in three parts:
(a) upper C7–T4
(b) middle T5–10
(c) lower end T10–L1

As has been mentioned in Chapter 6, the lower thoracic joints can, for the purpose of treatment, be regarded as part of the lumbar spine. The lowest two ribs which have no anterior attachment do not often require treatment unless there is abnormal tension in the quadratus lumborum muscle. If present this should be treated.

Simplified treatment using diagnosis by motion loss and muscle tension

Mid Thoracic Spine
(A) Supine technique described for stiffness of the T6–7 joint
with maximum muscle tension on the right side. (Fig. 60)
High Velocity:
    1 The patient lies supine with her elbows fully flexed and her fingers laced together behind her neck. It is important that the hands are very low on the neck in order to avoid

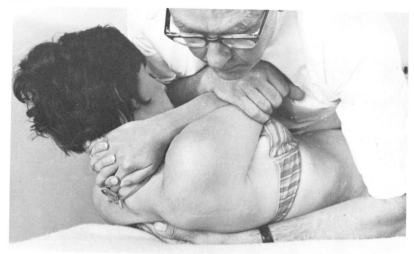

(a)

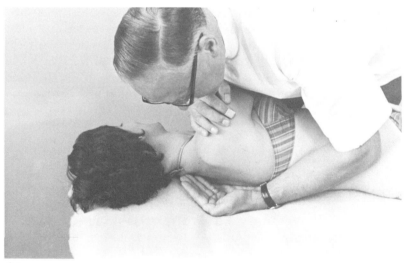

(b)

Fig. 60 (a) Supine treatment of mid thoracic spine. (b) The position in which the left hand is held.

uncomfortable hyperflexion of the head on the neck.

2 You stand facing her left side.
3 Grip her right arm just above the elbow with your right hand and roll the top half of her body towards you.
4 Introduce your left hand between her trunk and the table top in such a position that the tubercle of your

scaphoid bone contacts the transverse process of T7 (the bone below the level of the joint to be treated). Your thumb should point craniad and lie along the right paravertebral muscles. The spinous processes lie in the hollow of the metacarpophalangeal joints while the tips of your fingers support the left side of her spine.

5 Roll her back onto your left hand so that she is once again supine.

6 With your right hand and forearm lift her head and shoulders by pushing her elbows caudad thus flexing her spine from above down to the point that you begin to feel motion with your left hand.

7 Have her breathe in and then deeply out.

8 The thrust is given by leaning your chest over your right hand and her elbows and giving a high velocity low amplitude thrust with chest and right hand in the direction of your left carpal scaphoid.

NOTE:

(1) This is a hybrid technique, the elbows and locked upper spine being a long lever. The transverse process contact is a short lever.

(2) The manipulation produces gapping, flexion and a small amount of right rotation at the T6–7 joint.

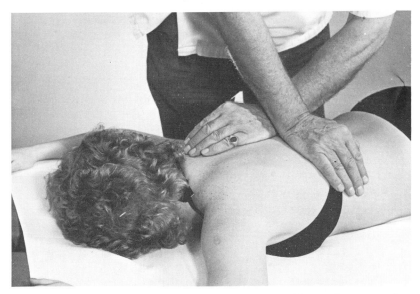

Fig. 61 Prone technique for mid thoracic spine with maximum tension on the right.

(B) Prone technique described for stiffness at T6–7 with maximum muscle tension on the right side. (Fig. 61)

High velocity:

    1 The patient lies prone with her head turned to the right.

    2 You stand at her right side.

    3 With your left pisiform bone contact the inferior aspect of the right tranverse process of her T6. Your fingers should point craniad.

    4 With your right pisiform contact the left transverse process of T7.

    5 Have her breathe in and then deeply out.

    6 At the end of the exhalation give a *short* thrust with both hands simultaneously. The thrust with the right hand should be downward (that is anteriorly with respect to the patient). That with the left hand should be craniad and anteriorly.

NOTE:

    (1) This is a short lever technique and although some force is required the distance travelled is small. The actual joint movement is less than an eighth of an inch.

    (2) This technique produces extension at the T6–7 joint and rotates T6 to the left. Because the contact with your left pisiform is on the caudal aspect of the transverse process of T6, the thrust also sidebends that vertebra to the left.

    (3) Because of the thoracic kyphosis the direction of the force with the lower (in this example right) hand should vary with the level; at about T6–7–8 it will usually be vertically downwards. Above that there ought to be a caudad component and below it a craniad component. The precise direction will depend on the shape of the individual curve.

    (4) Careful control of force is essential. Especially in the elderly it is possible to crack a rib if excess force is used.

    (5) This technique can be used in the lowest thoracic and even the upper lumbar joints.

(C) Sitting technique described for stiffness of the T6–7 joint with maximum muscle tension on the right. (Fig. 62)

High velocity:

    1 The patient sits on a stool or on the table with her legs over the side.

    2 You stand behind her.

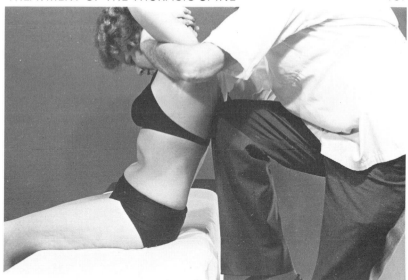

(a)

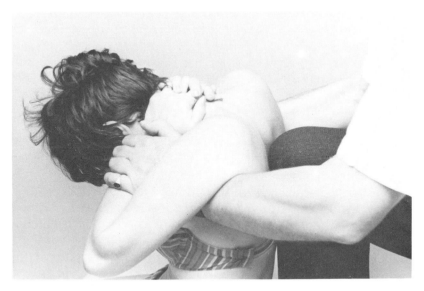

(b)

Fig. 62 Sitting technique for the mid thoracic spine. (a) With your hands on her neck. (b) With your hands on her wrists. (c) Using your abdomen as fulcrum.

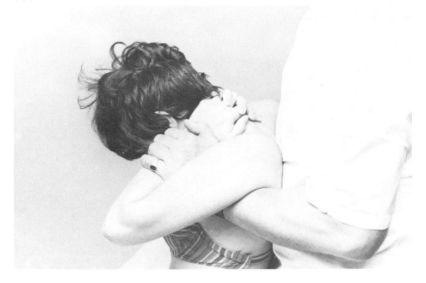

(c)

3   Put your arms through her axillae and bring your hands
    behind her neck lacing your fingers together. It is an
    advantage if she can put her hands over the back of
    yours, or
3a You instruct her to flex her elbows and lace her hands
    behind the back of her neck. You then thread your hands
    through her axillae and grasp her wrists.
4   You place one of your knees in her back to act as a
    fulcrum. This requires a support of suitable height for
    your foot. Sometimes the table (or stool) top will do.
    Often a lower support is required and a suitable stool
    may be used or a cross bar on the stool on which she
    sits. The height of the point of contact is critical. It
    needs to be at the level of the lower vertebra (T7 in this
    example). With the maximum tension on the right side
    the point of contact of the knee should be to the right
    in the region of the transverse process. If you have bony
    knees a small pillow between the knee and the patient
    makes her more comfortable.
5   You adjust the amount of flexion or extension at the
    T6–7 level by moving the patients' upper trunk with
    your arms. The tension should be felt to accumulate at
    that level.
6   Have her breathe in and then deeply out.

7   The manipulation consists of a short sharp pull with your arms upwards and backwards.

NOTE:

   (1) If the operator is moderately obese the upper abdomen can be used as a fulcrum but it is more difficult to make the level specific.

   (2) If you are using your abdomen as a fulcrum, the manipulation can be done standing.

   (3) By using different degrees of flexion of the upper spine the manipulation can be done in extension or in flexion.

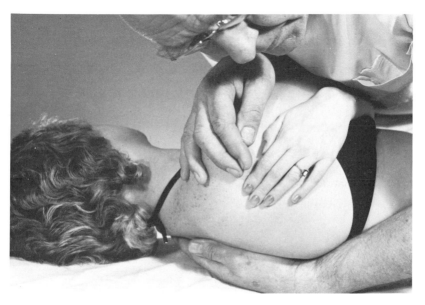

Fig. 63 Supine technique for upper thoracic spine.

Upper Thoracic Spine

(D) Supine technique for stiffness of the T2–3 joint with maximum muscle tension on the right side. (Fig. 63)

High Velocity:

   1   The patient lies supine.

   2   You stand facing her left side.

   3   Cross her arms over her chest. Her left arm should be next to her chest with her elbow in the midline and the right elbow lying over the top of the left elbow.

   4   With your right hand lift her right shoulder and roll her partly towards you.

   5   With the tubercle of your left scaphoid contact the right

transverse process of T3 and let your thumb lie parallel to the spine. Your hand should be slightly cupped with the fingertips supporting the left side of her spine and the spinous processes lying in the groove on the front of the metacarpophalangeal joints.

6 Roll her back onto your hand.

7 Produce forward flexion and some left rotation of the upper trunk by lifting her right shoulder with your right hand and pulling caudad and to the left until the tension accumulates over your left thumb (at the T2 level).

8 The manipulation is performed by a quick thrust given by your chest and right arm, at the end of exhalation through her arms and chest, in the direction of your left carpal scaphoid.

NOTE:

If too much force is used the costo-chondral junction of the 2nd right rib may be "sprung". This will cause pain that may last for about three weeks.

(E) Prone technique described for stiffness at the T2–3 joint with maximum muscle tension on the right side. (Fig. 64)

High Velocity:

1 The patient lies prone.

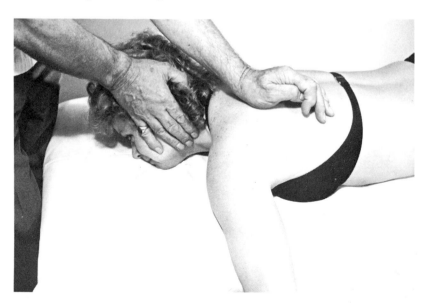

Fig. 64 Prone technique for upper thoracic spine.

2 You stand at her head.

3 Extend her neck so that her head rests on the table on her chin.

4 Place the pisiform of your right hand in contact with the right transverse process of her T3 vertebra.

5 With your left hand pivot her head to the left on the chin (thus producing rotation to the right and sidebending to the left) until the tension accumulates at the T2–3 joint. This can be detected by your right hand.

6 Have her breathe in and then deeply out.

7 The manipulation is performed by a short sharp increase in the pivoting movement with the left hand and a slight downward (anterior) thrust on the transverse process with your right pisiform.

(F) Sitting technique for C7–T1 (sometimes even for T1–2).

This technique is described in Chapter 9 under the heading "Typical Cervical Joints", treatment (A) high velocity.

Specific treatment using the results of positional diagnosis

Mid Thoracic Spine

1 *For dysfunction with neutral (Type 1) mechanics.* (Sidebending and rotation to opposite sides and spine in partial flexion).

Diagnostic points:

1 Several vertebrae rotated (treat the most rotated first).

2 Side bending restriction is to the side opposite to the rotation restriction.

3 Rotation is most marked in neutral and may disappear in full flexion or extension.

(A) Isometric treatment described for T6 rotated to the right: (Fig. 65)

1 The patient sits on the table with her legs over the side.

2 You stand behind her with a wide stance.

3 Control her trunk movement with your left arm. Reach through her left axilla and across her front to grasp her right shoulder. She should grasp her own left shoulder with her right hand.

4 Contact the right transverse process of T6 with your right thumb.

5 Bring up the tension under your right thumb by a combination of extension, right sidebending and left rotation of her upper trunk. Do not go beyond the point of tension.

6 Have her try to straighten herself against your unyielding resistance and then relax.

7 Take up the slack to the new tension point (barrier).

8 Repeat steps 6 and 7 two or three times.

NOTE:

(1) Left sidebending or right rotation can be used as the main corrective movement or it may be better to use a combination.

(2) If on re-examination there remains rotation at another level, that may also need treatment.

(3) An alternative grip may be used in step 3. You can reach under her left arm and grasp her right arm while she puts her right hand behind her neck and holds her right elbow with her left hand.

(B) High velocity treatment described for T6 rotated to the right: (Fig. 65)

1 The patient sits on the table with her legs over the side.

2 You stand behind her with a wide stance. Preferably position yourself in such a way that you can support your right elbow with your right hip in order to complete the thrust.

3 You control her trunk movement with your left arm.

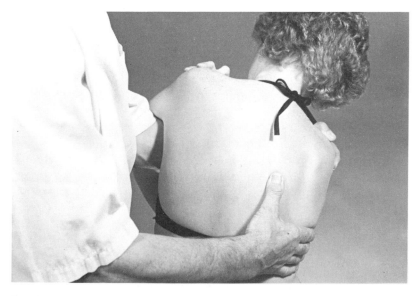

Fig. 65 Sitting technique for T6 rotated to the right in neutral flexion.

Reach through her left axilla and across her front to grasp her right shoulder. She should grasp her own left shoulder with her right hand.

4 Contact the right transverse process of T6 with the base of the thenar eminence of your right hand (compare Fig. 59).

5 Bring up the tension under your right hand by a combination of extension, right sidebending and left rotation of her upper trunk.

6 The thrust is given by a short sharp lifting force with your right thenar eminence in a direction that is anterior, craniad and to the left. This will make T6 move. T7 is stabilized by the weight below.

NOTE:

For an alternative grip at stage 3, see note 3 to technique A above.

2 *For dysfunction with non-neutral (Type II) mechanics.* (Sidebending and rotation to the same side and the spine either extended or well flexed).

(C) Isometric treatment described for a flexion restriction at the T6–7 level with restricted sidebending and rotation to the left: (T6 rotated to the right). (Fig. 66)

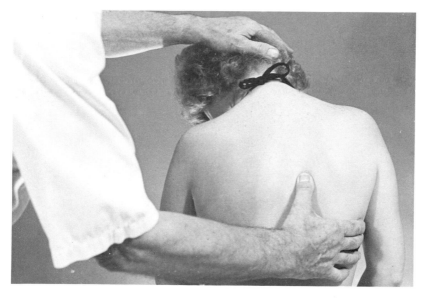

Fig. 66 Sitting technique for T6 rotated to the right with restricted flexion.

1 The patient sits on the table with her legs over the side.
2 You stand behind her.
3 You make local contact at the lesion.
   Either,
   (a) With your left thumb on the left side of the spinous process of T6.
   or,
   (b) With your right thumb on the right transverse process of T6.
4 Place your free hand on the top of her head.
5 Allow her to "slump" while guiding her head into forward and left sidebending. These movements are controlled precisely to the point where the tension can be felt to localise under the thumb contact at the T6 level.
6 Have her attempt to raise her head against your unyielding resistance and after a few seconds relax.
7 By adjustment of the amounts of flexion and left sidebending engage the new barrier.
8 Repeat steps 6 and 7 two or three times.

(D) Isometric treatment (with high velocity variant) for an extension restriction at the T6–7 level with restricted sidebending and rotation to the left: (Fig. 67)

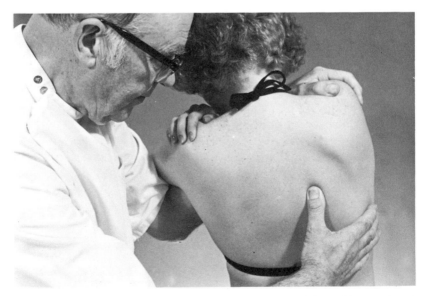

Fig. 67 Sitting technique for T6 rotated to the right with restricted extension. (Position after step 9.)

1 The patient sits with her legs over the side of the table.
2 You stand behind her.
3 You make local contact at the lesion with your right thumb on the right tranverse process of T6.
4 Reach through her left axilla with your left hand and grasp her right shoulder. She should grasp her left shoulder with her right hand.
5 With your left arm and hand sidebend her to the right in neutral flexion and rotate her to the left (see note).
6 Have her try to rotate her upper trunk to the right against your unyielding resistance.
7 Relax and take up the rotatory slack.
8 Repeat steps 6 and 7 twice.
9 Now, maintaining the rotation sidebend her to the left and have her push forward her abdomen to secure extension.
10 Have her attempt to flex and sidebend to the right against your unyielding resistance.
11 Relax and take up the slack in extension and left sidebending.
12 Repeat steps 10 and 11 two or three times.

NOTE:
  (1) If desired local contact can be made with your left thumb on the left side of the spinous process of T6. You then grip her left shoulder with your right hand and her arms are reversed.
  (2) This technique uses Type I mechanics for the first part because it is easier to restore the rotation by this means. Type II mechanics are used from step 9 on.
  (3) Instead of isometric treatment at step 10 a thrust may be used (compare technique B).
(E) High velocity treatment for a flexion restriction at the T6–7 level with limitation of rotation and sidebending to the left: (See Fig. 60)
1 The patient lies supine.
2 You stand to her right facing her.
3 Have her lace her fingers together low down behind her neck and bring her elbows together in front.
4 With your right hand grasp her right arm just above the elbow and rotate her upper trunk towards you. Place your left hand on her back so that the right transverse process of T6 is supported by the tubercle of your scaphoid. Your thumb should point craniad along the

right paraspinal muscles. Your fingers support the left paraspinal muscles and the spinous processes fit in the hollow of your hand.

5 Roll her back onto your left hand.

6 Introduce left sidebending by moving her head and upper trunk to the left.

7 With your right hand lift her shoulders by pressing caudally on her elbows in such a way as to induce flexion and left rotation of her upper trunk until the tension accumulates at T6. This is monitored by your left thumb. Be careful to maintain the left sidebending.

8 Lean your chest over your right hand onto her elbows and have her breathe in and then deeply out.

9 The thrust is given at the end of exhalation by a sudden short downward pressure by your chest and right hand on her elbows in the direction of your left scaphoid.

NOTE:

(1) Correction of this problem requires left sidebending given by the head and neck position and a combination of flexion and left rotation produced by the final positioning. The thrust increases both flexion and rotation.

(2) It is important that her hands should be low down on the neck. If they are high the head will be hyperflexed on the neck which is painful.

(3) This is a hybrid technique with one short lever by which movement of T7 is blocked, and one long lever through which the thrust is given.

(4) This is a more specific variant of the technique described under simplified treatment technique (A), (p. 133).

Upper Thoracic Spine

For lesions of the upper thoracic spine with neutral (Type I) mechanics.

The example given is for treatment of a T3–4 joint that will not sidebend to the right or rotate to the left.

Diagnostic points:

1 In both flexion and extension the thumbs on the transverse processes of T3 appear level and at the same depth.

2 In the mid range of sagittal plane motion the right transverse process is more posterior than the left.

3 The motion is not smooth.

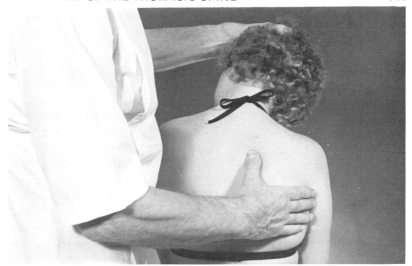

Fig. 68 Isometric technique for T3 rotated to the right in neutral flexion.

(F) Isometric: (Fig. 68)

Technique:

    1 The patient sits on a stool or with her legs over the side of the table.

    2 You stand behind her.

    3 With your right thumb contact the right transverse process of T4.

    4 With your left hand on her head you adjust the amounts of right sidebending and left rotation until the tension accumulates under your right thumb. This should be done in "neutral" flexion.

    5 Have her attempt to sidebend left and rotate right against the unyielding resistance of your left hand on her head.

    6 After relaxation take up the slack in right sidebending and left rotation until you reach the new barrier.

    7 Repeat steps 5 and 6 two or three times.

(G) High velocity: (See Fig. 64)

Technique:

    1 The patient lies prone.

    2 You stand at her head.

    3 Lift her head with your left hand, sidebend a little to the right and rest the head on the chin. With your left hand pivot the head on the chin to rotate the head to the left and increase the right sidebending. This movement is monitored by the right hand on the left side of her T3–4

joint and should not go beyond the point when tension rises at that joint. Alteration of the amount of side-bending may be necessary and is produced by moving the position of the chin on the table top.

4 Contact the cranial aspect of the left transverse process of T4 with your right pisiform.

5 The thrust is given by a simultaneous pressure caudally and anteriorly on the transverse process of T4 and a slight increase in the rotation-sidebend produced by pivoting the head.

For lesions with Type II (hyperextended or hyperflexed) mechanics.
For extension restrictions:

The example given is for treatment of a T3–4 joint that will not extend fully and will not sidebend or rotate to the right. (T3 rotated to the left).

Diagnostic points:

1 On flexion through the T3–4 level both thumbs ride up equally when placed over the transverse processes.

2 On extension the left thumb on the left transverse process of T3 comes down and back fully, becoming prominent. The right thumb does not come down fully and remains less prominent.

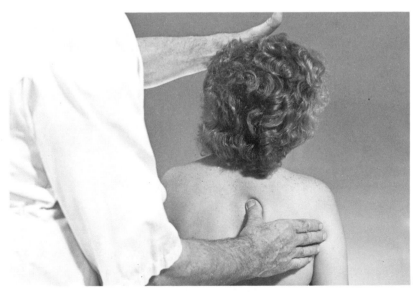

Fig. 69 Isometric technique for T3 rotated to left with restricted extension.

(H) Isometric Technique: (Fig. 69)
  1 The patient sits on a stool or with her legs over the side of the table.
  2 You stand behind her.
  3 With your right thumb contact the right transverse process of T4.
  4 With your left hand on her head you adjust the amounts of right rotation, right sidebending and extension until the tension accumulates under your right thumb.
  5 Have her attempt to flex, rotate left and sidebend left against the unyielding resistance of your left hand. For this purpose your left hand should, at this point, be holding the left side of her forehead.
  6 Have her relax fully and stop your pressure without losing your control of her position.
  7 After full relaxation take up the slack in extension, right sidebending and right rotation until you reach the new barrier. This will be indicated by the accumulation of tension once again under your left thumb.
  8 Repeat steps 5, 6, and 7 two or three times.
(I) High velocity technique: (Fig. 70)
  1 The patient lies prone.

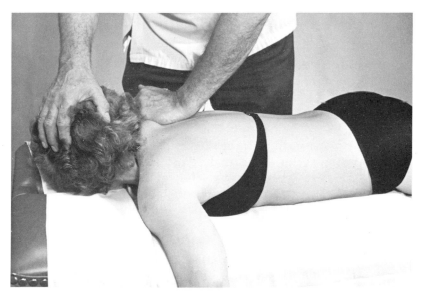

Fig. 70 Thrusting technique for T3 rotated to left with restricted extension.

2 You stand to her right.

3 With your right hand lift her head slightly, sidebend and rotate it to the right. Monitor the movement with your left hand and stop when the tension accumulates at the T3 level. Rest the head on the left side of the chin and maintain the position by your right hand on the right side of the back of her head.

4 Contact the caudal side of the right transverse process of T4 with your left pisiform bone.

5 Have her breathe in and deeply out.

6 Thrust with your left hand craniad and anteriorly while you slightly increase the pressure with your right hand.

NOTE:

The upward and forward thrust causes left sidebending and left rotation of T4 with the opposite reaction at T3–4 because T3 is controlled by locking from above.

For flexion restrictions:

The example given is for treatment of a T3–4 joint that will not flex fully and will not sidebend or rotate to the right.

Diagnostic points:

1 On flexion the left thumb on the left transverse process of T3 does not ride up or become less prominent. The right thumb moves up and forward normally.

2 On extension both thumbs ride down and back equally.

(J) Isometric Technique: (Fig. 71)

1 The patient sits on a stool or with her legs over the side of the table.

2 You stand behind her.

3 With your left thumb you contact the left transverse process of T4.

4 With your right hand on her head you adjust the amounts of right rotation, right sidebending and flexion until the tension accumulates under your left thumb.

5 Have her attempt to extend, sidebend left and rotate left against the unyielding resistance of your right hand. This time your right hand should be on the back of the left side of her head.

6 Have her relax fully and stop your pressure without losing your control of her position.

7 After full relaxation take up the slack in flexion, right sidebending and right rotation.

8 Repeat steps 5, 6 and 7 two or three times.

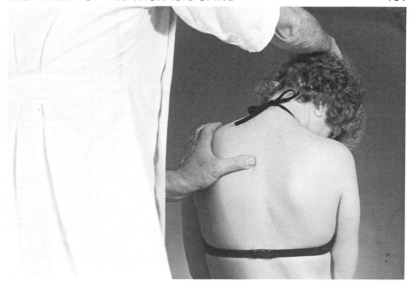

Fig. 71 Isometric technique for T3 rotated to left with restricted flexion.

(K) High velocity technique: (See Fig. 63)
    1 The patient lies supine.
    2 You stand facing her left side.
    3 Cross her arms over her chest. Her left arm should be next to her chest with her elbow in the midline and the right elbow lying over the top of the left elbow.
    4 With your right hand lift her right shoulder and roll her partly towards you.
    5 With the tubercle of your left scaphoid contact the lower part of the transverse process of T4. Your thumb should lie along the right side of the spine, the left side is supported by your fingertips.
    6 Roll her back onto your left hand.
    7 Produce right sidebending by side flexion of the neck.
    8 Grasp her right shoulder with your right hand pulling downwards and slightly to the left until you feel the tension accumulate at the metacarpophalangeal joint of your left thumb.
    9 Lean over your right arm with your chest and give a short thrust at the end of exhalation in the direction of your left carpal scaphoid with which you thrust cranially at the same time.

NOTE:
See note to simplified technique D, (p. 140) of which this is the more specific version.

TREATMENT OF RESTRICTED RIB MOTION

Disturbance of movement of the first rib will frequently accompany a C7–T1 or a T1–2 somatic dysfunction and these should always be treated before the rib motion is accepted as being abnormal.

There is some difference of opinion as to whether at other levels, the rib or the spine should be treated first. What matters more is that when one has been treated the patient should be re-examined and, if it is required, the other should then be treated. The author believes that treatment of the spinal joint first is usually preferable.

Exhalation restrictions

When treating exhalation restrictions the lowest restricted rib is the most important and should be treated first. Re-examination after such treatment will show if higher ribs also need to be dealt with.

Diagnostic points:

1 On exhalation one or more ribs stop moving before those on the opposite side.

2 There is usually restriction of motion in the corresponding spinal joint.

(A) Patient effort (ribs 2–10). Described for an exhalation restriction of the right seventh rib. (Fig. 72)

   1 The patient lies supine.

   2 You stand at the head of the table.

   3 Contact the upper edge of her right seventh rib with your right thumb so that it spans the costo-chondral junction.

   4 With your left hand lift her head and upper trunk until the tension reaches the seventh rib. If the rib dysfunction is predominantly of bucket-handle type, it is an advantage to introduce some sidebending to the right in addition to the flexion.

   5 Have her take a small breath in and then force it right out while you press the seventh rib caudad.

   6 Hold the rib down and take up the forward flexion and sidebending slack in the trunk.

   7 Repeat steps 5 and 6 two or three times.

   8 Have her extend her trunk and neck against your *yielding*

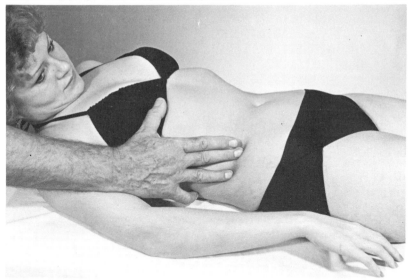

Fig. 72 Treatment of exhalation restriction of right 7th rib.

resistance while you maintain the rib position.

(B) Isometric (ribs 4–10). Described for an exhalation restriction of the right seventh rib.

    1 The patient lies supine.

    2 You stand at the head of the table a little to the right.

    3 Contact the upper edge of her right seventh rib with your right thumb so that it spans the costo-chondral junction.

    4 With your left hand lift her head forwards and sidebend her to the right until the tension reaches the seventh rib.

    5 Press her right seventh rib caudad to the barrier.

    6 Have her attempt to sidebend to the left against your unyielding resistance.

    7 Have her relax fully and stop your left hand pressure without losing the rib position.

    8 Take up the slack in the trunk position and in the rib.

    9 Repeat steps 6, 7 and 8 two or three times.

    10 Finally have her straighten her trunk against your *yielding* resistance while you hold the rib caudad.

(C) Isometric (ribs 2 and 3). Described for an exhalation restriction of the right third rib.

    1 The patient sits with her legs over the side of the table.

    2 You stand behind her.

    3 Hook the right index finger over her third right rib in

the axilla in order to pull it caudally.

4 With your left hand sidebend her head to the left and rotate to the left until the tension reaches the level of the third rib.

5 Have her attempt to straighten her head against your unyielding resistance.

6 Have her relax and stop your pressure on the head. As she breathes out assist the descent of the rib by keeping up the caudad pressure.

7 Take up the slack in the trunk position.

8 Repeat steps 5, 6 and 7 two or three times.

NOTE:

(1) Downward pressure on the ribs in the axilla is painful.

(2) If the restriction is mainly pump-handle in type the right index finger should be near the anterior axillary fold, if mainly bucket-handle it is better placed more laterally.

(D) Patient effort (rib 1). Described for right side exhalation restriction. (Fig. 73)

Diagnostic points:

1 The C7–T1 and T1–2 segments are functioning normally— after treatment if required.

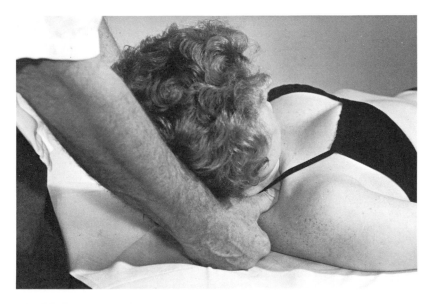

Fig. 73 Treatment of exhalation restriction of right 1st rib (elevated 1st rib).

2 On exhalation the right first rib stops moving before the left.

3 There may be loss of resilience to springing over the first rib.

Technique:

    1 The patient lies supine.

    2 You stand at her head.

    3 With your right thumb contact the front end of her right first rib behind the medial end of the clavicle.

    4 With your left hand flex her neck and upper trunk until tension accumulates under your right thumb.

    5 Have her take a small breath in and then breathe deeply out.

    6 As she breathes out assist the descent of the rib with your right thumb and take up the slack by increasing the flexion of the neck and trunk.

    7 Repeat steps 5 and 6 two or three times.

    8 Have her push her head back to the neutral position against your yielding resistance while you maintain the rib position with your thumb.

NOTE:

The anterior end of the first rib is always tender.

(E) High velocity (ribs 2–10). Described for a restriction of exhalation of the right fifth rib. (See Figs 60 and 63)

This treatment is very similar to that described for treatment of the thoracic intervertebral joints on page 139, treatment (D) for the upper thoracic spine. The difference is in the position of the fulcrum hand under the patient. Other high velocity techniques can similarly be modified to treat rib restrictions. Note the important but small difference between this and the high velocity method described for inhalation restrictions.

    1 The patient lies supine.

    2 You stand at her left side.

    3 You cross her arms over her chest—right arm uppermost —and left fingers in her right axilla.

    4 With your right hand lift her right shoulder and insert your left hand under her. Roll her back onto your hand in such a way that the tubercle of your left scaphoid contacts the inferior aspect of the angle of her right 5th rib. Your left thumb runs craniad along the right side.

    5 With your right hand pull her right shoulder caudad and to her left until the tension accumulates at your left carpal scaphoid.

    6 Lean over her and with your right arm and chest compress her chest in the direction of your left carpal scaphoid.

7 After a deep breath, at the end of exhalation, thrust by a sudden short increase in the downward pressure towards your left wrist.

NOTE:

(1) If there is more than one rib with an exhalation restriction treat the lowest first and then re-examine the higher ones.

(2) The manipulation tends to raise the angle and therefore to depress the front end of the rib into the full exhalation position.

(3) For the lower ribs the alternative technique described under treatment of the mid thoracic spine technique (A) on page 133, may be modified in the same way.

Inhalation Restrictions

If more than one rib has restricted motion, treat the uppermost first. If this is not done the upper rib will serve as a mechanical barrier to the full inhalation position of the rib immediately below.

The first rib may be very important but here it must be remembered that the function of the T1–2 segment should be checked, and if necessary treated, before a diagnosis of first rib dysfunction is made.

For isometric treatment of ribs with inhalation restrictions use is made of muscles that elevate the ribs.

For ribs 1 and 2 the scalenes are used, for ribs 3, 4 and 5 the pectoralis minor and for ribs 6 to 9 the serratus anterior.

(A) Isometric treatment described for inhalation restriction of the first or second right rib. (Fig. 74)

Diagnostic points:

1 The first thoracic vertebra moves normally on T2.

2 On inhalation the first rib on one side stops moving before that on the other.

Technique:

1 The patient lies supine.

2 You stand facing her left side.

3 With your left hand under her you curl the middle and ring fingertips around the first and second ribs near the transverse process and pull caudad and laterally.

4 With your right hand turn her head about 20 degrees to the left.

5 Place her right forearm across her forehead with the elbow at a right angle (see note).

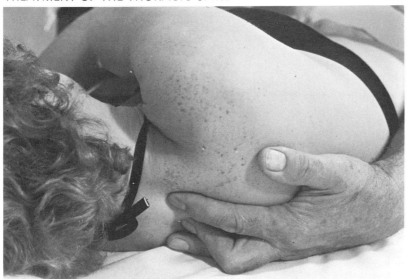

(a)

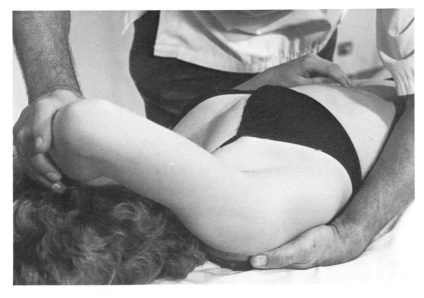

(b)

Fig. 74 Treatment of inhalation restriction of right 1st or 2nd rib. (a) The position of the under hand. (b) Position immediately before the isometric contraction. Note the position of the patient's right arm.

6 Hold her right forearm near the elbow with your left hand.

7 Have her breathe in deeply and then attempt to lift her head while you use your left hand on her right forearm to prevent movement.

8 Relax and then take up the slack with your right fingers.

9 Repeat steps 7 and 8 two or three times.

10 Bring her head back to neutral and release your finger pressure.

NOTE:

If she is unable to put her forearm across the forehead allow it to lie relaxed and use your left hand on her forehead for the counterpressure.

(B) Ribs 3–4–5.

Isometric treatment described for an inhalation restriction of the right 3rd, 4th, or 5th ribs. (Fig. 75)

Technique:

1 The patient is supine.

2 You stand to her left facing the head of the table.

3 Insert your left hand under her and hook the tips of the

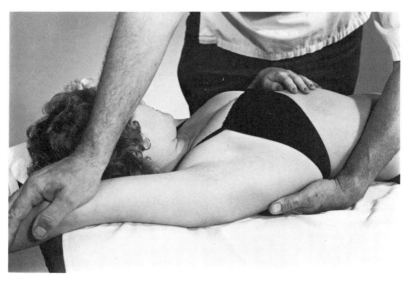

Fig. 75 Treatment of inhalation restriction of right 3rd, 4th or 5th ribs. Again note the position of the patient's right arm.

index, middle and ring fingers over her right 3rd, 4th and 5th rib angles.

4 Have her lift her right arm straight above her shoulder (see note below).

5 With your left hand pull caudally and laterally on her right ribs, concentrating on the one that is the uppermost of the restricted group.

6 Have her take a breath in and then attempt to bring her right arm forwards against the unyielding resistance of your right hand.

7 Relax. Take up the slack with the fingers of your left hand.

8 Repeat steps 6 and 7 two or three times.

9 Have her return her arm to her side and then remove your left hand.

NOTE:

If she is unable to raise her arm above her shoulder, the counterforce may be applied against her right coronoid process by your right thumb or thenar eminence. If this method is used it is important to take out the slack fully before the isometric effort is made. The effort she should make is to pull the coracoid caudally and to the left in the direction of the left breast.

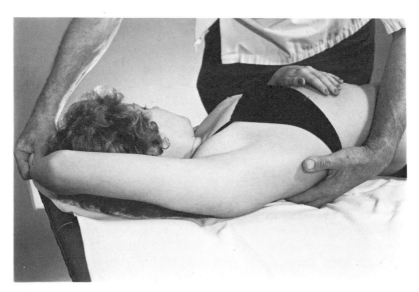

Fig. 76 Treatment of inhalation restriction of right lower ribs. Again note position of patient's right arm.

(C) Ribs 6–7–8–9.

Isometric treatment described for inhalation restriction of the right lower ribs. (Fig. 76)

Technique:

1 The patient is supine.
2 You stand to her left facing the table.
3 Insert your left hand under her and hook the tips of your four fingers over the angles of her right 6th, 7th, 8th and 9th ribs.
4 Have her elevate her right arm flexing the elbow so that the forearm lies above her head. (See note (2) below).
5 With your left hand pull caudally and laterally on her right ribs, concentrating on the one that is the uppermost of the restricted group.
6 Have her take a breath in and then attempt to bring her right arm to her side in the coronal plane. This you prevent by pulling on her right wrist with your right hand.
7 Relax. Take up the slack in the ribs with your left fingers.
8 Repeat steps 6 and 7 two or three times.
9 Have her return her arm to her side and then remove your left hand.

NOTE:

(1) This technique mobilizes all 4 of the lower rib group.
(2) If she is unable to put her right arm in the required position the counterforce may be applied by your right hand reaching over, grasping the scapula by the vertebral border and pulling it forwards and up. The effort should then be an attempt to bring her shoulder back against your resistance.

(D) High velocity. Described for an inhalation restriction of the right 5th rib. See Figs. 60 and 63.

1 The patient lies supine.
2 You stand at her left side.
3 You cross her arms over her chest as described for exhalation restriction.
4 With your right hand lift her right shoulder and insert your left hand under her. Roll her back onto your hand in such a way that the tubercle of your left scaphoid contacts the *superior* aspect of the angle of her right 5th rib. Your left fingers should support the left side of her spine and your thumb runs craniad along the right side.

5 With your right hand pull her right shoulder caudad and to her left until the tension accumulates at your left carpal scaphoid.

6 Lean over and with your right arm and chest compress her chest in the direction of your left carpal scaphoid.

7 At the end of inhalation the corrective thrust is given by a sudden short increase in this downward pressure coupled with a twist of your left wrist to thrust downwards on the angle of the seventh rib.

NOTE:

(1) If there is more than one rib with an inhalation restriction treat the highest first and then re-examine the lower ones. Treat if necessary.

(2) The manipulation tends to depress the angle and therefore raise the anterior end of the rib.

(3) For the lower ribs see the alternative referred to in Note 3 under exhalation restrictions technique (E).

9
Treatment of the Cervical Spine

Because of the great difference in structure and mobility between the atlanto-occipital, atlanto-axial and the remaining cervical joints a variety of techniques is required.

Almost the only serious accident to be reported following a treatment by manipulation has followed high velocity treatment in the upper neck. This is spasm with or without thrombosis in the vertebral artery or one of its branches. There is no record of such an accident with isometric treatment.

Atlanto-Occipital Joint

Diagnostic points:

1 Restricted motion between the mastoid process and the lateral mass of the atlas on sidebending the head.
2 Unequal translatory movement of the head on the body (treat the side opposite to that toward which translation is restricted). Note that at the atlanto-occipital joint rotation is always to the side opposite to that of the sidebend. The amount of rotation is very small.

(A) Isometric treatment described for a left sidebending restriction: (Fig. 77)

   1 The patient lies supine.
   2 You stand at her head.
   3 You hold her head between your hands monitoring atlanto-occipital movement with your index or middle fingers.
   4 Introduce left sidebending up to the barrier. When it is found that the restriction is most marked in flexion, the treatment should be carried out in flexion. When most marked in neutral or extension choose that position in the sagittal plane.
   5 Instruct the patient to attempt to sidebend her head to the right while you resist without yielding.

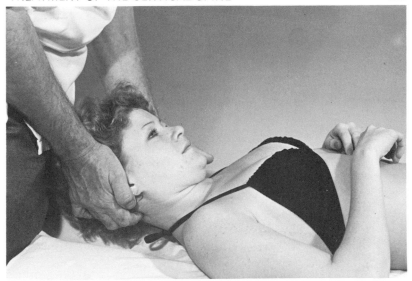

Fig. 77 Isometric technique for left sidebending restriction at the atlanto-occipital joint.

    6 Both relax. Take up the slack up to the new barrier when she has relaxed fully.

    7 Repeat steps 5 and 6 two or three times.

(B) High velocity treatment for a left sidebending restriction: (Fig. 78)

    1 The patient lies supine.

    2 You stand at her head.

    3 Contact the back of the right lateral mass of her atlas with your left index finger by sliding it transversely under the head. The left middle finger is placed with its pulp over the nail of the index finger to add support. This is done with the head flexed on the neck.

    4 Hold her chin with your right fingers and with your palm in contact with her right cheek.

    5 Take up the slack by sidebending left and rotation right until the barrier is reached and the tension can be felt to rise with the left index.

    6 The thrust is given by a high velocity, low amplitude increase in sidebending and rotation with the right hand against the resistance of the left fingers which are held still.

(C) High velocity treatment for a right sidebending restriction:

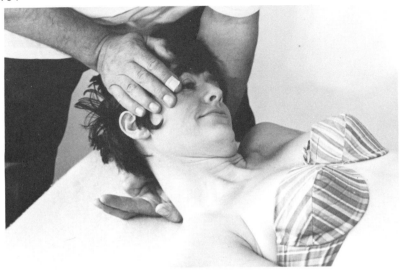

(a)

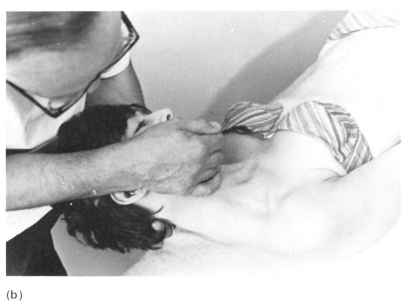

(b)

Fig. 78 (a) The "supported" left index finger. (b) Thrusting technique for left sidebending restriction at the atlanto-occipital joint.

For those sufficiently ambidextrous the mirror image of (B) can be used. Some will prefer: (Fig. 79)

1 The patient lies supine.
2 You stand at her head.
3 Contact the back of the left lateral mass of her atlas with your supported left index finger.
4 Grip her chin with your right fingers as in Technique B.
5 Take up the slack by sidebending right and rotation left.
6 Thrust with a high velocity low amplitude increase in the sidebending and rotation against the stabilized left side of the atlas.

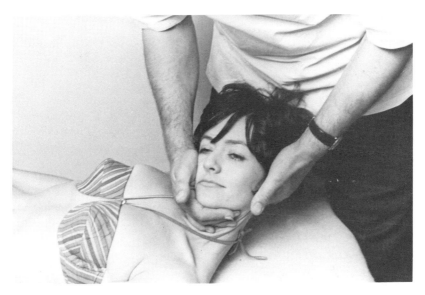

Fig. 79 Variant of thrusting technique for a right sidebending restriction.

Atlanto-Axial (C1–2) Joint

(A) Isometric treatment for left rotation restriction: (Fig. 80)

1 The patient is supine.
2 You stand or sit at her head.
3 Hold her head between your hands with index (or middle) finger in contact with the lateral mass of her atlas on each side.
4 Flex her neck to limit rotation in the lower joints.
5 Rotate her head to the left up to the barrier—as detected by the tension under the fingers. Do not sidebend.

6 Instruct the patient to rotate her head to the right against your unyielding resistance.
7 Both relax, take up the slack to the new barrier when she has relaxed fully.
8 Repeat steps 6 and 7 twice or three times.

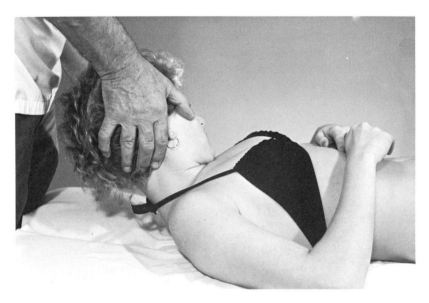

Fig. 80 Treatment of left rotation restriction at the atlanto-axial joint.

(B) High velocity treatment:
  See description of sitting technique (A) for lower cervical joints.

Typical Cervical Joints (C2–C7)
Treatment using diagnosis by motion loss and muscle tension:
Diagnostic points:
1 Loss of movement.
2 Muscle tight over the back of facet joint.
(A) High velocity treatment, described for stiffness of C4–5 with tight muscles on the right: (Fig. 81)
    1 The patient sits with her legs over the side of the table.
    2 You stand facing her and a little to her left.
    3 Reach around the right side of her neck with your left middle finger and contact the left side of the spinous process of C4. Squeeze forward on the articular pillar of C4 with the middle phalanx of the same finger.

4 Grasp the left side of her head with your right hand and by a combination of sidebending to the right, rotation to the left and, usually, extension the upper cervical joints are locked so that the force is concentrated at the C4–5 joint.
5 The joints below C5 are locked by the flexion produced by the forward pull of your left hand.
6 The thrust is given by a sudden short rotatory movement. Both hands are used to rotate the head and upper cervical vertebrae to the right thus carrying the C4–5 joint through the barrier that has been reached by the positioning.

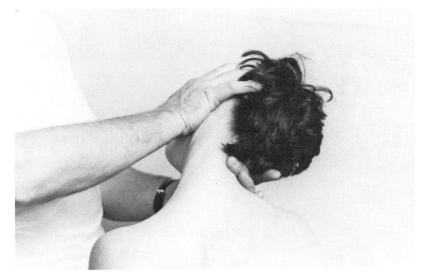

Fig. 81 Thrusting technique for cervical 4–5 with maximum tension on the right side.

NOTE:
(1) In the lower joints the finger is not long enough to reach the far side of the spinous process, it is therefore applied to the dorsal part of the articular pillar.
(2) This technique can be used for the C1–2 joints and often also for the C7–T1 and even T1–2.
(3) The index finger may of course be used and can be supported by the middle finger with the pulp closely applied to the index nail.

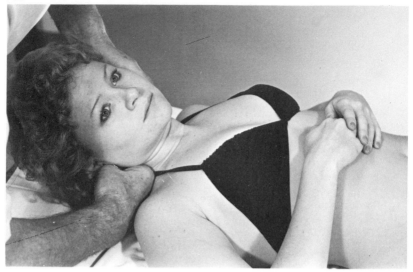

Fig. 82 Thrusting technique for restriction of right sidebending and rotation in neutral flexion.

Treatment using the results of positional diagnosis
(B) High velocity treatment described for restriction of right sidebending and right rotation at C3–4 in neutral flexion: (Fig. 82)
   1 The patient lies supine.
   2 You sit at her head.
   3 Support her head with your left hand.
   4 Contact the right articular pillar of C4 with the lateral side of your right index finger.
   5 Lift her head slightly, sidebend over your right index finger and rotate to the left enough to bring the tension to the level of the right index.
   6 Perform the correction by a high velocity, low amplitude thrust with the right index in the direction of the left orbit. There is, of course, a simultaneous tightening of the position by the left hand.

NOTE:
   As described the thrust moves the lower vertebra C4 on C3. If it is desired to move C3 on C4 the index finger should contact the articular pillar of C3 and the thrust must then be downwards and backwards toward the tip of the spinous process of C7.

(C) Isometric treatment described for restriction of flexion and sidebending-rotation to the right (left facet opening restriction) at C4–5: (Fig. 83)

1 The patient lies supine. You stand at her head.

2 You cradle her head between your hands using your fingers to palpate the C4–5 facets. Your finger on the left side should support the articular pillar of C4.

3 Sidebend and rotate her head to the right in flexion adjusting amount of each movement until tension under the palpating left fingers indicates engagement of the barrier.

4 Maintain the position by pressure of the left hand and instruct her to push against your hand.

5 Both relax. Take up the slack to the new barrier when she has fully relaxed.

6 Repeat two or three times as required.

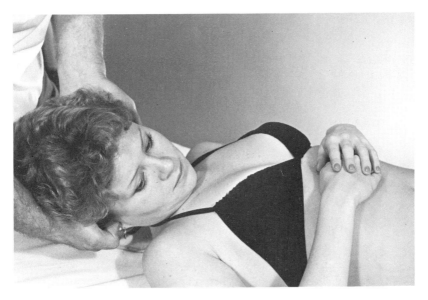

Fig. 83 Isometric technique for restriction of right sidebending and rotation at C4–5 with restriction of flexion.

(D) Isometric treatment for restriction of extension and sidebending-rotation to the left (left facet closing restriction) at C4–5: (Fig. 84)

Treatment in flexion can be used with the addition of a final

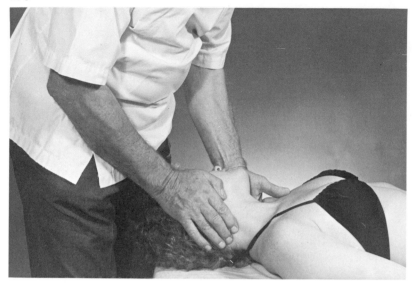

Fig. 84 Isometric technique for restriction of right sidebending and rotation at C4—5 with restriction of extension.

isometric extension correction, but note that the sidebending rotation is now reversed. Or,

1 The patient lies supine. You stand at her head.
2 You cradle her head between your hands using your fingers to palpate the C4—5 facets. Your finger should support the articular pillar of C5 on the left side.
3 Sidebend and rotate her head to the left in extension adjusting each movement until tension accumulates under your palpating finger on the left side.
4 Move your right hand to the right side of her forehead and instruct her to lift her head against your unyielding right hand.
5 Both relax. Take up the slack to the new barrier when she has fully relaxed.
6 Repeat two or three times as required.

NOTE:

For extension restrictions the finger should be on the bone below the joint being treated.

Sitting Isometric Techniques

For the lower cervical joints the sitting techniques described for the thoracic spine may be used. See Chap. 8 techniques H and J. (Figs. 69 and 71)

10

The Plan of Treatment

In previous editions of this book, this chapter opened with the following sentence, "The working hypothesis is that the pathogenesis involves stiffening of one or more intervertebral joints probably resulting from damage and associated with local muscle spasm." With further experience and in particular with experience of other manual methods of obtaining relief, my thinking has altered. In this connection I would like to add that I am under no illusion that my present thoughts are likely to be final.

The isometric contraction techniques described in this book cannot be expected to force a joint to move beyond the range which is easy. By virtue of the nature of these techniques it seems clear that they act on muscle not joint. There are other techniques, which I have not attempted to describe, which can also achieve success, but in which no external force is applied to the patient whatever. These are known as indirect techniques and are very useful in the acutely ill patient if treatment is needed. These techniques depend on observation of muscle tension and very careful alteration of position to produce the minimum tension in the area. It is difficult to see how this kind of simple positioning could have any effect on a mechanical upset in the joint. The relaxation of muscle can be felt to happen.

It is now my opinion that the basic problem is one of a muscle that becomes too tight and will not relax.

To be more precise, the problem appears to be that of over-action of the gamma motor neurone system which becomes self-perpetuating. The effect of this is to shorten the resting length of the muscle. If this shortening persists the muscle cannot return to its normal resting length. Shortening produced in this way is of course physiological. Shortening of the resting length is required prior to certain types of action of muscle, particularly those in which anything near the maximum power needs to be exerted through a short range. It is a quite different phenomonen from that of cramp which appears to be a total contraction of the entire muscle. When the resting length is shortened the muscle is still able to contract further and then to relax back to where it was. It appears that the pain is produced in some way by its inability to relax to its full resting length.

If this hypothesis is correct, it follows that the limitation of joint movement is a result of the muscle tightness and not the cause of it. What a pity that the so-called muscle relaxants all seem to be cerebral depressants rather than to have any direct effect on muscle. If some chemical could be found which had a selective effect on the gamma system it might be more helpful, even if it upset the general postural tone of the body.

This hypothesis immediately poses a question. If the problem with which we are dealing is pain arising from tight muscle, why does manipulation of the joint help? The question only arises with treatment by high velocity manipulation. Isometric muscle contraction has been known for many years to help secure relaxation.

It appears that the effect of a high velocity manipulation is to use the bones involved in the joint as levers to stretch the tight muscles. This would also explain the importance of doing the manipulation in the right direction.

Experience with manipulative treatment shows that it is rarely sufficient to mobilize the affected joint on one occasion only. The muscle appears to behave as if there were a built-in memory in the neuromuscular unit so that it tends to go back to its contracted state, even when it has been stretched. From the standpoint of neurophysiology there does not appear to be any reason why the neuromuscular unit should not have a memory of this kind. The number of treatments required varies very much from patient to patient. The factors which tend to increase the number are the length of time for which the lesion has been present, the severity of the violence which produced it, the frequency of further similar strains in the course of daily life, and the state of emotional tension of the patient. The latter will be discussed later.

In some patients it is found that the first few manipulations produce a temporary increase in soreness and sometimes also in the total amount of pain. Fortunately in such cases there is usually some sign of improvement, most commonly an increase in mobility. A common reason for inadequate improvement following treatment by manipulation is that there has been failure to find the most important joint. Precise diagnosis is not easy. It can become even more difficult if, as a result of overtiredness or for some other reason, the manipulator's sensory perception is not at its best. Errors in precise localization of the lesion are not uncommon even for experienced manipulators. Errors can be of two different kinds. First, a true error. For whatever reason the precise localization of the signs was incorrect and the wrong joint was treated. Secondly, a joint was treated which was of secondary importance only and the symptoms persist (or even can be aggravated) because the primary joint is still causing trouble. In a patient with pain arising from the low back there may well be loss of movement and soft tissue changes at the T12–L1 joint; and, indeed, treatment of that joint may be required before the condition is fully resolved. It may be, however, that this same patient has limitation of movement and soft tissue changes in the neighbourhood of the sacro-iliac joint. If the sacro-iliac joint happens to be the primary cause, treatment of the upper level will at best result in temporary partial improvement. Treatment of the sacro-iliac joint, however, if it is primary, can even result in resolution of the problem at the upper joint.

The importance of a full structural diagnosis has been alluded to in an earlier chapter. These considerations make it important that on each occasion one should perform a further examination at least in the areas where abnormality was previously found. This in turn is the author's reason for preferring always to do the actual manipulative treatment himself rather than to delegate it to a medical auxilliary.

There is however, another common cause of persistence of pain in spite of proper manipulative treatment. This is the existence and persistence of secondary areas of painful muscle spasm. These areas used to be known as fibrositis and when the term was restricted to that meaning it was a useful one. They are most commonly found in the gluteal region and in the muscles around the scapula. In this connection it is proper to define what is meant by the use of the word spasm in the this context. It is meant here to refer to the same type of persistent loss of extensibility probably due to overaction of the gamma system. These areas in peripheral muscle are associated with specific patterns of referred pain. Much of the original work on this subject was done by Travell[1]. These patterns have been reproduced recently by Mennell[2] and he also describes Travell's technique of combining muscle stretching with the application of cold to the overlying skin.

Even a superficial study of the diagrams in Mennell's paper

will show that the referred pain does not follow recognized patterns of nerve distribution. There seems to be little doubt that many of these pain sources in peripheral muscle themselves result from a disturbance of nerve function caused by spinal joint problems. Other possible causes have been suggested by Wyke whose work is discussed in Chapter 11.

Travell lists common sites for such trigger points:

1 producing pain in the low back; the quadratus lumborum or the longissimus dorsi;
2 producing pain in the lower limb; the glutei, the adductor group;
3 producing pain in the neck and head; the sternomastoid, the trapezius, the suboccipital muscles, the muscles of mastication;
4 producing pain in the shoulder; the trapezius, the levator scapulae, the scaleni, the posterior cervical muscles;
5 producing pain in the arm; the spinati, the scaleni, the deltoid, the subscapularis, the pectoralis major and minor.

In addition the pyriformis should be mentioned as being an important muscle which is often associated with loss of function in the sacro-iliac joint on the same side. This muscle is not easy to feel and is therefore easy both to forget and neglect.

In a special review of muscle pain syndromes Simons[3] gives an excellent review of the extensive literature on the subject. According to his review Reichart in 1937 was the first to associate explicitly the three classical features; (1) a point of exquisite tenderness within (2) a circumscribed palpable hardening of muscle, and (3) pain referred in response to pressure on the tender point. Travell's first paper on trigger points appeared in 1942 and she has published many subsequent papers. Mennell (*loc. cit.*) has drawn most of her material together in his recent paper which includes many of her charts of pain reference from the trigger points. Simons quotes many authors who failed to find histological or serological evidence of abnormality in biopsy specimens removed during surgery. Only in severe long-standing cases was there some fibroplasia. In his conclusion Simons points out that "only in the last several decades has this distinction between trigger zones and reference zones been drawn clearly and distinctly." He also finds that "several lines of evidence have suggested that something interfered with the oxidative metabolism of muscle fibres in the region of a palpable band." Reference to the charts published by Mennell will show that in a few instances the trigger point lies within the zone of referred pain. This of course increases the likelihood of confusion between the two areas.

Although the precise nature of the changes which cause the thickening and the exquisitely tender point are not firmly established, there can be no doubt in the minds of clinicians that these painful areas in muscle do exist. Most people who treat this kind of pain will know of patients in whom treatment of the trigger zone resulted in complete relief of the pain. Unfortunately this is not usually what happens. More commonly, there is temporary relief followed by a return of the pain and when the pain returns it will usually be found that the trigger point has once again become active.

It seems likely that the trigger point in peripheral muscle is itself started by a disturbance of function of its nerve supply, probably the gamma system. One of the causes of such disturbance of the nerve supply is an interference with normal function of one or more joints in the spine. If treatment of the trigger point results in lasting relief it appears reasonable to assume that the original exciting cause is no longer active. If after treatment of a trigger point there is temporary relief followed by recurrence it may well be that the exciting cause is still active. Patients coming for treatment of pain should always be checked for trigger points but a positive finding does not necessarily complete the diagnosis. It is probably a commoner mistake to neglect the muscle trigger points and treat the spinal condition; it can be equally unsatisfactory to treat the trigger point and neglect the spine.

There is one further importance of trigger points which underlines the necessity for finding and treating them. This is that a persistent trigger point appears to be able to cause a recurrence of the abnormal muscle tension in the spinal muscle which initiated the trigger point in the first place. The mechanism seems to be that the pain producing afferent discharge which maintains the trigger point is capable of overflowing to affect the spinal muscles, much in the manner in which the spinal muscle problem initiated the peripheral trigger point.

For the sake of simplicity the word fibrositis will be used to signify an area of abnormal tightness in peripheral muscle fibres often, but not always, having within it the true trigger point as defined by Travell.

A remarkable property of referred pain is that it can appear to be exactly the same, when produced by either of two (or more) separate sources. It will be a familiar experience to most manipulators that occasionally the secondary fibrositic areas have been neglected while the primary manipulative treatment of the spine has been continued. This can lead to a state when the spinal lesion itself has settled but the secondary fibrositic areas are maintaining the symptoms in almost identical form. Treatment of the fibrositic areas themselves at this stage can result in a very dramatic recovery. The known occasional effectiveness of treatment of fibrositic areas without any spinal treatment is probably dependent on the same phenomenon, the spinal joint lesion having settled enough to stop being a direct cause of symptoms before treatment was undertaken.

The treatment of the fibrositis can, of course, be undertaken by a physiotherapist, but fortunately the majority will settle relatively easily, provided that the exciting cause is also treated. The exciting cause is usually a spinal joint lesion and it is commonly practicable for the manipulator to treat the fibrositic areas at the same time as he treats the spinal joint lesion. Other sources of segmental pain can produce the same reaction.

Various types of treatment are available. Of these, perhaps the simplest is the application of heat. Heat in any form will do, but dry heat is as good as any and easier to apply. The infra-red lamp is a good method of applying radiant heat but this appears to have no particular advantage over contact heat from a hot water bottle or an electric hot pad. The last two have the advantage that they are equally effective when applied outside the clothing. In order to use an infra-red lamp, removal of clothing is necessary and, unless one is careful, it is easy to burn the skin. This treatment, of course, the patient can do for herself at home. It is helpful but not usually curative.

Massage has been used for many years but in order to be effective the treatment must be given deeply. This is often acutely painful and can easily become intolerable. It must be started gently and the fingers are gradually worked in more deeply. Frictioning with the thumb can be used but it is usually better if the tips of the fingers are worked across the muscle bundles in an attempt to stretch out their contracture.

The feeling of an area of fibrositis is quite characteristic. Part of the muscle involved is thickened and feels tight to the fingers while the neighbouring areas are normally soft (and painless). The thickened muscle has aptly been termed "cordé" and feels much as if the bundles were a series of tight cords. It gives the impression that these fibres are in a chronically contracted state.

The result of successful massage of this kind proves that they are not fibrosed because, when relaxation is obtained, the fibres once again feel like normal muscle. This can sometimes be achieved in a very short space of time.

If one does not start the treatment gently, the patient will often refuse to allow it because it becomes too painful. Treatment of this kind starting gently and working in deeply enough is time consuming and tiresome, but can be very important. If the area is so sensitive that no effective stretching can be given to the muscle fibres, the attempt should be abandoned. In some such cases deep frictioning with the thumb may be helpful but in many it is better to resort to infiltration of the muscle area.

For such infiltration, the author's practice now is to use local anaesthetic (1 per cent lignocaine). For some years he used a freshly prepared mixture of lignocaine 2 per cent in equal parts with hydrocortisone (25 mg in 1 ml) but the mixture does appear in some people to produce a reaction which is unpleasant. (The mixture must be freshly prepared, because the addition of local anaesthetic solution causes the hydrocortisone suspension to precipitate.) The experience of many colleagues in this field encouraged the author to go back to plain local anaesthetic and the results have been very satisfactory in the majority of patients.

For the occasional patient who does not respond to local anaesthetic alone, the author still uses the hydrocortisone-lignocaine mixture. Soluble synthetic steroids can be obtained in stable, sterile mixture with local anaesthetic. They are convenient but the author prefers the less potent but effective hydrocortisone. Steroids alone can be used especially in those sensitive to the local anaesthetics.

In this connection, Travell has obtained similar results with dry needling of the trigger points, although it seems likely that for dry needling the trigger point itself must be more accurately delineated. It is interesting to speculate as to whether the relief of trigger point muscle spasm, and the referred symptoms which it can cause, might bear any relation to acupuncture. The beneficial effects of Rees-Seely Rhizolysis are probably due to direct trauma causing relaxation of trigger point muscle spasm.

Travell and others[2, 4, 5] have developed a technique of obtaining relaxation of the muscle spasm using a vapo-coolant spray. For this purpose, ethyl chloride was originally used, but it was found that a mixture of freons had better physical characteristics without the dangers of anaesthetic effect or inflammability. The technique is to put the affected muscle on the stretch while spraying with the cooling liquid over the corresponding area of skin.

This technique has now been used by many people over a period of years and there is no doubt from the author's personal experience that it is often most effective. Mennell[2] gives a summary of much of the work done both by Travell and himself and has an excellent series of diagrams showing the trigger points and their reference zones. He also describes in detail the treatment with vapo-coolant spray. A similar skin chilling can be produced by the use of ice. Dr. Audrey Bobb (personal demonstration) uses an ice cube for the purpose and using fairly firm pressure moves the ice cube transversely across the area of the trigger point thus producing both temporary cooling and some stretching of the muscle fibres. Unfortunately, this has two disadvantages. (1) The patient gets wet. (2) It is a lot more painful than the use of vapo-coolant spray. Prolonged cooling should be avoided. It has been known for many years that prolonged chilling will make these areas worse.

If, in spite of injection treatment, the fibrositic areas continue to recur it is a sure sign that the exciting cause has not been relieved.

Similar treatment is sometimes required for the areas of muscle spasm in more immediate relationship to the damaged joint. This is particularly so in the very acute case in which it is impossible to position the patient adequately for the manipulation to be performed.

Here again the most effective treatment is massage given transversely across the fibres of the muscles which are running up and down the spine. It may be given with the tips of the fingers from either side or with the heel of the hand, in which case the operator should stand on the side opposite the lesion, because a pushing movement away from the midline is easiest with the heel of the hand. Once again it is important to start gently in order to prevent overstimulation and resulting pain and fresh muscle spasm.

Injection treatment is also possible but rather larger quantities are required and the use of steroid preparations seems less justified.

An alternative method of securing relaxation of the spinal muscles in the area of the joint lesion is by the use of a caudal epidural injection of local anaesthetic. This can also give lasting relief of pain in some patients. For these purposes, this injection can be given satisfactorily through the sacral hiatus and by this route, requires no special preparation. For lesions in the low thoracic region larger quantities are required but for the common low lumbar lesions, 20 ml is nearly always enough and this figure can be reduced for the small patient. The injection is best given with the patient lying prone and if the pain or flexor muscle spasm prevents the adoption of this position, enough pillows should be used to support the abdomen to allow her to lie in relative comfort. The lateral position can be used but is less convenient for the operator.

There is no need for a preliminary injection to anaesthetise the skin. The use of a sharp disposable needle of adequate length for the full injection causes no more pain in the skin than the tiny hypodermic needle which is sometimes used as a preliminary. The sacral hiatus is found and the needle introduced in the midline pointing upwards (craniad) and forwards, the angle required usually being about 30° to the horizontal. It is easy to feel when the needle has pierced the tough fibrous tissue which covers the sacral hiatus and if it is correctly placed, it will then advance without further obstruction for a centimetre or two. Usually the injection will flow relatively easily but it is uncomfortable and remains so until it has ceased, in spite of the action of the local anaesthetic. The discomfort is described as a heaviness in the region of the sacrum itself or as an exacerbation of the pain in the leg. The latter complaint is comforting to the operator who knows that the injection is in the correct place. The injection must be given slowly and if the pain becomes intense, it is better to stop for a short time to allow it to settle before finishing. It is always wise to perform an attempted aspiration before making any injection. This serves to prevent the accidental injection of the solution into the spinal theca or intravenously. There is no need to use a long needle and if one of no more than $1\frac{1}{2}$ in is used, the danger of an intrathecal injection is almost non-existent. Local epidural injections can be used by those familiar with the technique and are much better for lesions above the lowest thoracic joints. For these it is of course essential to be certain that the dural sac is not entered.

After the injection, the patient is allowed to lie in any comfortable position for a few minutes until the local anaesthetic takes effect. If the injection is successful, at the end of this time it will be found that the pain is partially relieved and that the muscle spasm has become less. The operator can then proceed with the necessary manipulation with an enhanced likelihood of success.

It is always wise to arrange that the patient will not drive herself home after such an injection. If the quantity is restricted to 20 ml and the strength is not more than about one-half per cent of Lignocaine (or similar local anaesthetic) it is unusual for any serious weakness of the legs to develop. In the occasional patient, however, there is a transient major weakness which would make driving unsafe and which even makes it difficult to walk from the car into the house. The patient must be warned of this and it will be readily understood that the rate of diffusion is such that it is more likely to happen at the end rather than at the beginning of the patient's journey home. This effect will wear off in the course of a few hours but, unless the patient has been warned, it may lead her into danger as well as cause her great alarm. If local epidural injections are given higher up it is wise either to do this in hospital, or to provide facilities for the patient to rest for $1\frac{1}{2}$ to 2 hours before going home.

Unfortunately spinal joint lesions are not commonly single. In those who are suffering from their first injury to the spine there may well be only one joint showing stiffness. The majority of those who come for treatment, however, either give a history of an injury some time before and of many attacks, or give no history of injury at all. In these the primary strain may have occurred so long before that it has been forgotten. In such people one usually finds stiffening of several joints and it is important that those which have muscle spasm over them should be treated. The secondary stiffened joints will commonly be found either at the next joint above or below that which appears to be the cause of the main symptoms, but more distant joints can also be affected. In the lumbar region it is relatively common to find one of the sacro-iliac joints affected. A consideration of the mechanics will show that if the lumbo-sacral joint has become stiffened in such a way that the body of the 5th lumbar vertebra is rotated to the right relative to the sacrum, the left sacro-iliac joint is likely to be in the position with the innominate posterior relative to the sacrum. This is the position in which the joint most commonly becomes stiffened. From any primary lumbar lesion, it is not uncommon to find secondary stiffness in the low thoracic region, at the cervico-thoracic junction or in the upper part of the cervical spine. These same levels are also found to be vulnerable for development of secondary joint stiffness when the primary injury is other than in the lumbar spine and the reason is probably to be found in that these regions are the junctions between parts of the spine of different function and different mobility. This change of character appears to cause an increased susceptibility to injury.

Treatment of a Patient with a Possible Disc Protrusion
In the absence of signs indicating a space occupying lesion it can
be very difficult to distinguish between a patient with an actual
disc protrusion and one with very acute symptoms from a spinal
joint lesion without this complication. Experience with manipulative treatment suggests that there is no single clinical sign and
no combination of signs that prove diagnostic other than those
of a space occupying lesion. The severity of the pain is no guide
nor is the immobility of the spine nor the presence of a scoliosis
nor the degree of limitation of straight leg raising nor the
alteration in the straight leg raising test caused by dorsiflexion
of the foot. The spinal joint lesion in which disc damage is
sufficient for bulging to have started appears to be made no
worse by the type of manipulation described in earlier chapters.
The results of manipulation, however, are often much less good
in such cases. The actual manipulation, therefore, can be used as
a diagnostic test to be continued only so long as improvement
occurs.

There is no doubt that some cases with actual disc protrusions
do improve with manipulative treatment. This improvement
however, is noticeably slower than the usual. In such cases it
can still be worth proceeding with manipulations but it is wise
to assess each individual case on its merits and to explain in detail
to the patient what the diagnosis is and what the alternative
treatments are. If the situation is explained to them, many such
patients will elect not to have surgery if there is any reasonable
alternative and, provided continuing improvement does take
place, some of those will prefer to continue with manipulation
rather than submit to immobilisation either by continuous
traction or by a plaster jacket or brace. If treatment is persisted
with for long enough, even those cases in which a true disc
protrusion is diagnosed will often settle very satisfactorily
without the need for surgery.

Chrisman et al.,[6] report on a series of 38 patients suffering
with "an unequivocal clinical picture of a ruptured intervertebral
disc unrelieved by conservative care". Twenty seven of these
had positive myelograms. All were submitted to rotatory manipulation under anaesthetic and 20 are reported as having good
or excellent results. Ten of those with positive myelograms
remained good or excellent three years or more after manipulation. The appearance of the myelogram before and after the

manipulation, whether positive or negative, was unchanged. They did note, however, that the results were better in the group with negative myelograms. An example of a case with a positive myelogram is given in the appendix (Case 37).

Frequency of Treatment

The advisable frequency of treatment in any particular patient will depend on a number of factors. Obviously it is undesirable to continue treating so frequently that any reaction produced by the manipulation is not allowed to settle between treatments. On the other hand, if treatment is insufficiently frequent, progress may become so slow as to be non-existent. In hospital out-patient practice it is not often easy to arrange for treatment more frequently than at weekly intervals. Experience suggests that an interval of one week is probably more efficient than a longer interval, but two weeks is acceptable for the less acute cases and for those patients who have already received the major part of their treatment. When possible, daily treatment for the first few days appears to be the best for the acute case. The danger of a build-up of soreness from inflammation or other results of manipulation is real, however, if one continues to treat the patient at daily intervals for any period of time.

Most patients can, with advantage, be treated three times a week until the acute phase is over. Treatment is then tailed off fairly rapidly to twice and then once per week or even less frequently. The number of treatments required by any particular patient varies enormously. Some are almost completely relieved by one treatment, others, particularly those of the more chronic type, require treatments repeated on many occasions in order to obtain lasting relief. The operator must be guided with respect to the frequency and the number of treatments by his findings on clinical examination. If it is clear that the patient is improving with respect to the extent and intensity of muscle spasm and the range of general and specific mobility, then the frequency of treatment can usually be decreased quite rapidly. The large majority of patients will admit to symptomatic improvement corresponding in extent and rate to the observed clinical change. In such patients, it is usually quite safe to allow one's views on frequency and length of treatment to be influenced by their subjective complaints.

The operator is well advised always to re-examine thoroughly any patient whose improvement is slow. One of the common causes of slow improvement is a failure to treat one or more of the areas of somatic dysfunction.

The Problem of the Neurotic Patient

It is well known that back trouble is often found in association with neurosis. This association has, in the past, proved a particularly tiresome one for the medical practitioner because he has not had an adequate yardstick by which to measure the actual disability caused by the back condition, nor is there any means of forming a quantitative assessment of the severity of a neurosis. This has undoubtedly led to unnecessary treatment for back complaints in patients in whom the back condition was minor and the neurosis severe. It has also led to the neglect of genuine back trouble in a great many patients who also have a neurosis. Indeed, it requires a very stable personality to avoid a neurosis when one is told by a supposed expert that one's back pain has no physical basis, however genuine it may feel.

Unfortunately, this situation is still all too common because the techniques necessary for detailed examination of the spinal column are either not known or not used. When such patients are positively diagnosed as having a physical abnormality, and when their pain is relieved by treatment, the improvement in their personality sometimes has to be seen to be believed.

The neurotic with a bad back can be a difficult problem. If the neurosis is an iatrogenic one produced by failure to diagnose and treat a genuine back lesion then it can be expected to settle so satisfactorily as to be no problem. Unfortunately, there are many patients who have a neurosis not basically the result of back trouble but who also have a back problem of greater or less severity. The patient who presents herself for examination and in whom there is almost no physical abnormality is relatively easy to deal with. One must, of course, take the trouble to perform a full, thorough examination in order to exclude not only back joint lesions of the type under discussion, but any of the other physical abnormalities that might cause such trouble. If one has successfully excluded physical causes, the patient should on no account be started on a course of manipulative treatment. Such patients are rare and the following example is a warning to be careful.

A man in his mid-thirties was admitted to an orthopaedic hospital at which, at the time, the author was a registrar. After exhaustive clinical and x-ray investigation he was discharged labelled a neurotic, although he was still complaining bitterly of his back. Three months later we heard from a neighbouring hospital that he was dead of leukaemia.

Among those sent for examination because of back complaints the neurotic without back trouble is a comparative rarity. It is much more common to find that even in a patient who appears to be seriously neurotic, there is physical evidence of back trouble requiring treatment. In some of these cases the neurosis is due to the back trouble and will respond dramatically to its treatment. Unfortunately in others the neurosis acts as a tiresome complicating factor which makes treatment considerably more difficult. These are the problem cases and it is idle to deny that they create a problem both in hospital and in private practice. The difficulty arises in two ways. First, by the very nature of their personality, they tend to feel pain more than those who are more stable and they also complain more loudly about it. Secondly, the increased nervous tension, which is an integral part of neurosis, reflects itself automatically in an increased muscular tension.[7] This in turn causes a relative increase in the abnormal muscle tension over the back joint lesions. In the severe neurotic this excess general tension can make it almost impossible to treat any underlying back trouble and such cases usually need psychotherapy in some form. In others, improvement can be obtained in the condition and, at the same time, the elementary psychotherapy which is the stock in trade of any good doctor, can be used to assist the patient. In some this may have an effect out of all expected proportion and, if nothing else, it does relieve the general practitioner temporarily of some of the load which these patients cause. The recognition of such cases is of great importance to the manipulator. If he fails to do so he is in danger of being "lumbered" with a high proportion of neurotics for whom his treatment is doing little or nothing, who clutter up his waiting-room and bring his practice into disrepute.

Dangers and Contraindications

There is scarcely a treatment in medicine that is without its attendant danger. There is the possibility of doing harm by almost any active treatment and this is certainly true of manipulation. Fortunately the dangers are small and with care they can be avoided. It is of the utmost importance, however, that they should be recognised.

These dangers fall into three groups:

1 those caused by the manipulation doing damage to a bone

weakened by some pathological process with possible dissemination of that process;
2 spinal cord or cauda equina pressure caused by massive disc extrusion;
3 circulatory disturbance caused by reflex arterial spasm.

Dangers in Manipulating a Weakened Bone

Bone is commonly weakened by one of a few pathological processes. All of these will in time be visible in x-ray pictures but patients may well be seen in the stage when the bones are already significantly weakened but the x-rays do not yet show any change. This is particularly true of infections and neoplasms. The most common cause of weakening of bone is osteoporosis and this is always detectable in the x-rays.

Clinical judgement is a vital part of the assessment of any candidate for manipulative treatment. The osteoporotic can nearly always be spotted from across the room if one has a "high index of suspicion". No such case should ever be manipulated without prior radiography.

Tuberculosis is fortunately much less prevalent than formerly. It remains a danger and one which must not be forgotten because of its comparative rarity. One should be put on one's guard at once because the patient is usually ill—as well as in pain. In infection the intensity of the muscle spasm over the lesion is much greater than one finds in the simple traumatic case. If one is unfortunate enough to manipulate a tuberculous lesion this muscle spasm proves to be a very helpful ally because, with the type of manipulation described in this book, it virtually prevents any movement at the affected level and therefore prevents harm being done. This is a good reason for never using general anaesthesia which abolishes the spasm.

Simple tumours of sufficient size to weaken the bone are uncommon in the vertebral column.

Primary malignancy is also uncommon but multiple secondaries are common and may cause serious loss of strength before they are visible in the x-ray. Fortunately the clinical picture usually points to some major general disturbance of body economy which arouses one's suspicions. This, however, is a good reason for refusing to see a patient unless sent with a history by her own doctor!

In discussing dangers one must not forget that the osteoporotic patient may well have a spinal joint lesion amenable to manipulation, so indeed may the patient with malignant disease.

Danger of Massive Disc Extrusion

This accident has occurred often enough to be the basis of serious argument against manipulation.

It happened to two of the author's patients. One merely stooped to lift a heavy article, the other sat up in bed and coughed. Both had been having manipulative treatment not long before the accident. Both had surgery but unfortunately recovery in the first was incomplete.

The only iatrogenic case of which the author has personal knowledge occurred when a spine was manipulated under general anaesthesia and the manipulation included forced flexion.

The type of disc degeneration that can predispose to massive extrusion is fortunately rare, the worst kind being that in which there is a separated calcified disc sequestrum. It appears that the accident is most unlikely to happen if anaesthesia is not used and if forced flexion is never performed. Both of those in the author's practice occurred from a self-imposed flexion strain.

If the accident does happen and cauda equina paralysis ensues exploration and removal of the disc material is essential and must be done without delay. Even a half-hour may be of vital importance.

Danger of Reflex Arterial Spasm

Theoretically one might suppose that this could happen at any level to the segmental arterial supply of the spinal cord. In practice the only accidents reported in recent literature involved the posterior inferior cerebellar artery or vertebral artery and have occurred with upper cervical manipulations only.[8]

These have all been in chiropractor's cases and in most of them there was evidence of arteriosclerosis with or without anatomical abnormality. The arterial spasm may be more frequent than is reported because it seems only to cause lasting symptoms when thrombosis follows. In that case cerebellar necrosis may occur and the outcome may be fatal.

Maigne[9] draws attention to the narrowing of the vertebral artery which occurs in some persons on positioning of the head and refers to arteriographic studies which sometimes demonstrate complete occlusion.

The literature does not show that positioning of the head produces occlusion in every patient but it strongly suggests that, in those who are at risk from manipulation, positioning will produce symptoms from circulatory embarrassment.

Tissington Tatlow and co-workers[10, 11] performed angiography on cadavers and found complete occlusion of one artery in 5 of 41 subjects with full extension of the head on the neck and rotation to 90 degrees. The occlusion was always in the artery on the side opposite to that to which the face was turned. When the examination was repeated with traction applied as well (amounting to half the body weight) 12 more subjects produced unilateral occlusion and 3 bilateral. They noted incidentally that in 3 of 41 subjects one vertebral artery was more than twice the diameter of its fellow. In the first paper an additional occlusion was shown at the level of C5–6 joint where there was a lateral osteophyte but all the other occlusions were at the atlanto-axial joint or above.

Sheehan and co-workers[8] observed that, in those suffering from symptoms due to spondylotic vertebral artery compression, rotation and hyperextension of the neck can produce comparable symptoms. They found however that the symptoms were produced by compression or occlusion at the sites of exostoses in the intraforaminal portion of the artery. They agree that physiological narrowing of the supra-axial portion occurs in all people on rotation of the head.

Bauer et al.[12] demonstrated changes in the electro-encephalogram on head turning in those with vertebral artery disease but only when carotid compression was applied as well.

It seems probable that the accidents were due to the occurrence of spasm in the vessel which, because of anatomical abnormality or disease, was carrying the greater part of the blood supply to the basilar artery. It also appears likely that the positional test will show up at least the large majority of those likely to be subject to such a complication at whatever site the narrowing occurs.

The test is very simple. The head is first extended as far as it will go and then rotated first to one side, then to the other. The position should be maintained for several seconds to allow symptoms to develop. These symptoms are likely to be dizziness, nystagmus or dysarthria.

The work of Tissington Tatlow et al.[11] suggests that traction can be dangerous, especially in combination with extension and rotation. It seems likely that, for the upper cervical spine, manipulation is better done with the head flexed rather than with it extended.

Excessive violence should always be avoided, particularly in this region.

The reported cases of reflex arterial spasm appear only to have occurred during manipulation of one or other of the upper two cervical joints. All appear to have been subjected to high velocity manipulation. It is worthy of note that both these two joints can easily be treated by isometric techniques without any violence. Many patients respond very well to this type of treatment. Unfortunately an occasional patient fails to respond adequately and in that case it may be necessary to consider high velocity manipulation.

Osteoarthritis

True osteoarthritis of the apophyseal joints is relatively uncommon and must be distinguished from degenerative disc disease. The hypertrophic spurs on the margins of degenerate discs are, of course, an attempt on the part of the body to restrict abnormal movement. Spines showing these changes will commonly respond satisfactorily to manipulative treatment. An example of a patient successfully treated by manipulation is shown in Fig. 67. In such cases the joints causing the symptoms are often found to be those not showing very marked changes.

In previous editions of this book a recommendation was made that patients with true osteoarthritis of the facet joints should be treated by some means other than manipulation and a support was recommended. Much further experience with such patients shows that in nearly all of them the symptoms are arising from a different level which will respond to manipulation and when this is not so even the osteoarthritic joint can be manipulated with relief.

The Problem of the Short Leg

The author's practice is to neglect leg length difference when the patient is first seen. This follows the belief that the patient has had the difference all her life and is partly compensated.

If the improvement in symptoms is delayed unexpectedly, or if recurrences occur in spite of successful treatment, a raise in the shoe may be prescribed.

It is usual to recommend a raise in the heel only unless the amount exceeds a half inch. The heel on the long leg side may, of course, be lowered.

The amount of the raise should always be a little less than the difference.

Movable lifts inside the shoe are not recommended.

Greenman[13] discusses the use of lift therapy in detail.

REFERENCES

1 Travell, J. and Rinzler, S. H. (1952), The myofascial genesis of pain, *Postgraduate Medicine* **11**, 425–434.
2 Mennell, J. M. (1975), The Therapeutic Use of Cold. *JAOA* **74**, 1146–1158.
3 Simons, D. G. (1975), Muscle Pain Syndromes. *Am J. Phys. Med* **54**, 289–311 and **55**, 15–42.
4 Travell, J. (1960), Temporomandibular joint dysfunction. *J. Prosthetic Dentistry* **10**, 745–763.
5 Travell, J. (1952), Ethyl chloride spray for painful muscle spasm, *Arch. Physical Medicine* **33**, 291–298.
6 Chrisman, O. D., Mittnacht, A. and Snook, G. A. (1964), A study of the Results Following Rotatory Manipulation in the Lumbar Intervertebral Disc Syndrome, *J. Bone Jt. Surg.* **46A**, 517–524.
7 Simons, D. J., Day, E., Goodell, H. and Wolff, H. G. (1943), Experimental studies on headache, *Res. Publ. Ass. Nerv. Ment. Dis.* **23**, 228–244.
8 Sheehan, S., Bauer, R. B. and Meyer, J. S. (1960), Vertebral artery compression in cervical spondylosis, *J. Neurol.* **10**, 968–986.
9 Maigne, R. (1968), *Douleurs d'Origine Vertebrale et Traitements par Manipulations*, Paris, Expansion Scientifique. p. 144.
10 Tissington Tatlow, W. F., Bammer, H. G. (1957), Syndrome of Vertebral Artery Compression, *Neurology* **7**, 331–340.
11 Brown, B. St. J., Tissington Tatlow, W. F. (1963), Radiographic Studies of the Vertebral Arteries in Cadavers, *Radiology* **81**, 80–88.
12 Bauer, R. B., Wechsler, N. and Meyer, J. S. (1961), Carotid Compression and Rotation of the Head in occlusive Vertebral Artery Disease. *Ann. Internal Medicine* **55**, 283–291.
13 Greenman, Philip E. (1979), Lift Therapy: Use and Abuse, *JAOA* **79**, 238–250.

11

The Intervertebral Joint Lesion

The precise nature of the changes which take place in an intervertebral joint causing it to start producing symptoms, are still the subject of argument and of many conflicting theories. As has been stated earlier, there appears to be one certainty, namely that there is no "little bone out of place". There are relatively few basic physical signs which can be elicited in a high enough proportion of cases, to justify the belief that they are fundamental to the condition. The natural history, the unsatisfactory results of surgery in some cases, and many other factors suggest that actual protrusion of disc material is a complication rather than the primary condition. The basic physical signs which can be established beyond reasonable doubt are:

1 loss of spinal mobility;
2 spasm in the musculature in the areas of the diminished mobility;
3 tenderness.

In the acute phase, the loss of mobility is widespread but when this is over, there remains a stiffness localised to one or more individual spinal joints. Owing to the ability of neighbouring segments to increase their range of movement and compensate for the stiffness of the damaged joint[1] there is often little or no loss of overall movement. If, however, further joints become stiffened, a loss of overall range is likely to develop. This individual joint stiffness can be detected both by clinical and x-ray means, but, for either, special techniques are required. These have been described in earlier chapters and it is essential that some technique of this kind should be employed before it is said that there is normal mobility in any section of the spine.

In the acute phase the muscle spasm is very obvious and no one will deny its existence. In the more chronic case this may also require careful examination in order that it is not overlooked. Examination for muscle spasm is much more difficult in patients who are grossly obese but it will also be found to be difficult in those people who have a particular type of subcutaneous tissue which appears to be more fibrous than the usual and through which it is considerably more difficult to feel.

Examination of the spine in patients who have a long history of symptoms arising from the back will usually reveal a number of levels that are not normal. Loss of movement at one level may be associated with increased movement at one or both of the neighbouring joints. This is more likely to happen where two or more joints together have lost part or all of their range of movement. This condition of hyper-mobility can be inferred sometimes from x-rays taken in the standard positions. This is most commonly seen in the cervical spine in patients who have severe degenerative change at more than one joint. In such a patient with, for example, marked narrowing and anterior spur formation at the disc spaces between C4–5, 5–6 and 6–7 the position of C3 relative to C4 may be so far flexed as to be almost a subluxation. (Fig. 85) These joints will usually be tender but detailed examination reveals increased mobility rather than loss of motion. High velocity manipulation is not appropriate treatment for such a joint. Even so, it may be possible to give relief to the neighbouring stiffened joints and take the strain off the hypermobile one. I think it is doubtful if high velocity manipulation would ever be justified for such a joint. It should be clear, however, that these negative considerations do not apply to isometric treatment.

In the presence of multiple joints with restricted mobility it can be difficult to find out, to start with, which are the most important. If the important joints are neglected the patient's progress will be a lot less satisfactory, although progress may still be made. Loss of mobility will be present in any joint which is a significant part of the overall problem. Tissue texture and tension changes are also likely to be present but they may well be most marked at the joints which are the immediate cause of current symptoms. Joints may be symptomatically silent, even when they are significant parts of the primary cause leading to the symptom complex of which the patient complains. At these levels the soft tissue changes are unlikely to be so marked. As has been mentioned before this constitutes the main reason for performing a general skeletal examination rather than confining one's attention to the localised area complained of.

In a patient who has had recurrent symptoms over a period of time it is usually possible to find abnormalities of vertebral

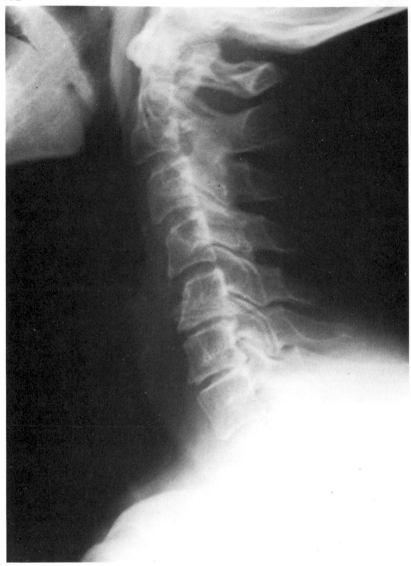

Fig. 85 Cervical spine showing narrowing and other degenerative changes at the C5–6 and 6–7 levels. Note the excessive forward projection of C4 on C5. In this case it is probably due to wearing away of the upper aspect of C5 by the movement occurring at the C4–5 level. This joint should be treated with caution and the appearance is a contraindication to high velocity treatment in that part of the neck.

position and usually soft tissue changes as well. If these are found it is likely that that the patient's liability to recurrence can be reduced by treatment. Before embarking on treatment for such a patient it is important to assess the economics of the situation. In such circumstances it would obviously be possible for the treatment to be of benefit to the manipulator's pocket-book more than to the patient.

The paucity of clinical signs and the diversity of the symptoms produced by spinal joint disorders confused the medical profession to such an extent that they were not always recognised as having their origin in spinal joints. The work of Mixter and Barr[2] stimulated interest in the intervertebral disc as a cause of referred symptoms. Since that time an immense amount of work has been done but it appears that many of the pieces of the puzzle are still missing. There can be no doubt that actual protrusion and extrusion of disc material occurs in some patients and can cause physical pressure on nerve roots or on the cord itself. Such protrusion or extrusion in fact produces a space occupying lesion in the spinal canal and may have to be distinguished from other such lesions. Even in this connection, however, there are a number of factors that require explanation.

First is the well-established but often forgotten fact that pressure on a nerve causes paralysis but no pain. An excellent example of this in the author's practice was a young man who had been sailing. In order to keep the boat on an even keel during a straight run lasting for more than half an hour, he leant against its side. Unfortunately, the main site of the pressure was immediately over the radial nerve as it winds round the humerus. When he moved, he found that he had a complete wrist drop and the pressure had continued for long enough for this to take between eight and ten weeks for full recovery. He was adamant that at no time had there been any pain.

It is probable that some types of stimuli to the dural investment of the nerve root can cause pain but the evidence in support of this does not appear to be conclusive.

Secondly, there is from time to time the unusual patient who demonstrates unequivocal signs of a disc protrusion with a disability due to stiffness and altered nerve conduction but who has almost no pain. These patients will often give a history of having had pain in the earlier stages and can be distinguished from those with congenital abnormalities of pain sensation by their response to other painful stimuli.

Thirdly, there is the observation that in many cases, symptoms of back and referred pain have been present for a long time before there is any evidence of an actual disc protrusion.

When a true protrusion is found, a careful evaluation of the history will often fail to reveal any dramatic change in symptoms until there is sufficient pressure on the nerve to produce the different signs of a space occupying lesion.

Charnley[3] was clearly unsatisfied that the disc was the primary cause of symptoms when he wrote, "One of the most surprising things about acute lumbago is that the amount of pain does not seem to be proportional to the amount of organic change visible in the disc. . . . We rarely find convincing protrusions in these cases, but what is cogent to the present argument is that the material removed appeared more often to be normal than fibrous and stringy."

Friberg and Hult[4] found symptoms of sciatica without detectable herniation of discs.

Pedersen, Blunck and Gardiner[5] considered that they had evidence that back pain and sciatica could arise from stimulation of sinuvertebral nerve fibres.

The old generations of medical manipulators commonly referred to the lesions as a fixation or a strain. Several modern manipulators have felt that the results of manipulation were attributable to some change in the intervertebral disc itself. Cyriax states in many of his publications that he believes that by his manipulations he actually reduces disc protrusions. Armstrong[6] gives diagrams of how he believes manipulation can influence a nuclear sequestrum (although he does go on to condemn manipulation in any form). Burke[7] believed that pain was due to erosion of the inner aspect of the posterior annulus by damaged elements of the nucleus and that manipulation would move the nucleus forward away from the sensitive point.

Anyone with experience in disc surgery will know that the nuclear material in a disc protrusion is not normal. Instead of being a firm jelly-like substance, it is composed of a softened sticky material which is somewhat stringy in consistency. From the anatomy of the disc we know that protrusion cannot possibly take place until a track is formed down which this nuclear material can be forced. There is no known blood supply to either nucleus or annulus of the disc except to the most superficial layers of the annulus. It is inconceivable that an almost totally avascular structure would be able in a few minutes to seal the track even if the protrusion itself had been withdrawn by a manipulation.

Nachemson and Morris[8] give recordings of pressure inside intervertebral discs and their figures vary from 50 to 80 kg/cm^2 when lying, through 90 to 120 kg/cm^2 when standing to 100 to 127 kg/cm^2 when seated. It seems unbelievable that, under a hydrostatic pressure of this magnitude, the softened nuclear material would remain in the nuclear space after it had been withdrawn there by a manipulation, when there was a preformed channel by which it could again protrude. These theoretical considerations would suggest that continuous traction would be more likely to be effective both in securing and maintaining reduction of a disc protrusion into the nuclear space. Traction is of course of considerable value in the treatment of patients and in particular, of those with acute back pain. There appears to be no evidence to suggest, however, that actual disc protrusions can be reduced by this means.

As has been pointed out in an earlier chapter, there are two joints in the spine itself which have no intervertebral disc but which can be the source of symptoms strictly comparable to those seen in joint lesions in other parts of the spine. Reference was also made to strains of the sacro-iliac joint as the cause of similar symptoms. It has been known for many years that sacro-iliac strain could be a cause of low back pain and there are many published records to show that dramatic relief could be given by manipulation.[9, 10] At the present time there is a general feeling (once shared by the author) of blank disbelief at the suggestion that any symptoms can arise from this joint, least of all symptoms of pain referred to a distance. This attitude appears to have arisen from the medical profession's general preoccupation with the intervertebral disc as the cause of symptoms and the belief that for the production of referred pain, actual pressure on nerves or nerve roots was required. There is of course, no nerve of any size on which pressure can conceivably be brought by a minor movement of the sacro-iliac joint. Documented instances in the literature concerning the symptoms produced by lesions at the atlanto-occipital and atlanto-axial joint, are much more difficult to find than are those concerning the sacro-iliac joints.

It is noteworthy that Cyriax[11] in the description of his techniques makes no reference to individual joints in the cervical region. There is no reference to the atlanto-occipital or atlanto-axial joint either from the point of view of production of symptoms or from that of treatment. He does describe techniques for manipulating the sacro-iliac joint but he does not describe the symptoms which can arise from it and he regards sacro-iliac lesions as rare. Examples from the author's practice of patients providing strong clinical evidence of symptoms arising from atlanto-occipital and sacro-iliac joints are given in a later chapter.

Injections of local anaesthetic sometimes produce effects which are difficult to explain on the theory that the pain is due to some change in the intervertebral disc itself with or without protrusion causing nerve root pressure.

The first is that occasionally, a patient is seen in whom areas of acutely tender fibrositis have arisen and in whom injection of these areas with local anaesthetic is followed by dramatic relief of symptoms not only of the pain in the area of the fibrositis but also of the back pain and referred leg pain which has been present. Even in those cases in which the relief is not dramatic or long-lasting, there is sometimes enough temporary relief of leg pain to confirm the impression that the area of fibrositis is acting as a secondary focus for the reference of pain. A somewhat similar effect can be produced by injection of local anaesthetic solution into the muscles and ligaments around a spinal joint causing symptoms.

The second is that, at least in some patients, the caudal epidural injection of a weak solution of local anaesthetic can be enough to abolish the pain before there is any effect either on the sensory or motor function of the nerve roots in the low lumbar region. Burke[7] suggested that the effect was on the nervi sinu-vertebrales of Luschka and he tried to explain the radiation of pain by a process of electrical induction. Unfortunately the induction theory does not stand up to critical examination.

Lindblom[12] and Perey[13] showed that when a needle is introduced in order to perform a discogram the posterior longitudinal ligament proves to be sensitive. The pain experienced is only severe if the disc is abnormal. When the needle is advanced into the nucleus no pain is felt. When the solution is injected a mild low back pain is produced if the disc is normal but in an abnormal disc which is not ruptured distension reproduces both the back pain and the sciatica. The remarkable finding is that this pain is still reproduced when the solution injected contains 1 per cent of novocaine.

Wyke's[24] recent work has been referred to in Chapter 2. He has shown that there are three routes by which pain fibres reach the dorsal root ganglion. All three consist of fine fibres either with very thin myelin sheaths or with no sheath at all. It seems reasonable to suppose that any of these fibres would be affected early by a weak solution of local anaesthetic in the epidural space. It is tempting to think that an abnormal discharge of impulses in one or more of these nerves could be one of the exciting factors in the production of symptoms.

Wyke also points out that these nerve endings can only be caused to discharge by either mechanical or chemical irritation. He considers that mechanical irritation can arise from:

1 abnormal postural stress;
2 local oedema, either due to direct trauma or acute inflammation;
3 direct compression;
4 excessive distension of the veins in the paravertebral plexus.

Chemical irritation causing pain can result from:

1 irritants associated with inflammatory exudates;
2 much less commonly, iatrogenically.

According to Wyke, stimulation of these pain receptor systems causes reflex contraction of related muscles and, if such spasm be sustained, it itself will give rise to chemical irritation of the receptor endings, closing the circle. In this way, muscular pain is superimposed on and may become more important than the primary spinal pain. Wyke also reminds us that reflex spasm produced by a painful visceral lesion can likewise start a spinal pain-spasm-pain cycle which is self-perpetuating.

The problem of referred pain is one which has received much attention from neurologists, anatomists and physiologists. Kellgren[14] reports work started by Lewis and carried on by himself in which an irritant solution of 6 per cent saline was injected into volunteers at various sites. He showed that by injecting the irritant beside the spinous process of the 1st sacral vertebra he could produce the typical pain of sciatica with radiation all down the leg. The injection was partly into ligaments and partly into muscles and possibly also into the periosteum over the sacral laminae. A similar injection at the level of the 1st lumbar spine produced a typical attack of lumbago. Similar work has been done by other workers[15, 16, 17] and a discussion of the results is given by Troup.[18] Many of the workers have noted that referred pain is associated with hyperalgesia of the area to which the pain is referred and this is commonly accompanied by a cutaneous hypoaesthesia. The evidence of the experimental work is said to suggest that there is not only a distal but also a central mechanism involved in the production of referred pain and the suggestion is made that the central mechanism is both in the higher centres and in the cord itself.

It appears clear that actual damage to the segmental nerve root is not necessary in order to produce referred pain. This pain need not be confined to the dermatome or the sclerotome of that level.[17]

The importance of the true disc protrusion must not be underestimated. The dramatic relief which often follows surgical removal of a large protrusion is very gratifying to both patient and surgeon. Unfortunately surgery for back pain is not always so satisfying and even in cases that are initially successful, acute recurrences can still occur. The author well remembers a bank manager in his middle forties who seven years previously had had a severe sciatica due to a disc protrusion which was removed at operation. The result was delightful until one week before, when the pain had begun to return, and very quickly got severe, although there had been no known injury. Fortunately he responded dramatically to manipulative treatment. Within four to five treatments he was again pain-free and the acute anxiety precipitated by the recurrence of the pain had completely subsided. When he was seen for this recurrence there were no abnormal neurological signs although straight leg raising was much reduced. There was no clinical evidence to suggest a true disc protrusion and the results of the treatment certainly did not suggest that there had been such a protrusion. The chief point of interest is that something fresh had happened in the lumbar spine which was amenable to manipulation but yet produced a recurrence of the symptoms previously relieved for a long period by removal of the disc at operation.

The changes in the intervertebral disc in those who have actual protrusions are accepted as being due to degeneration. The cause of this degeneration is unknown although by many it is assumed to be the result of trauma. Roaf[19] said, "Prolapse of a normal disc either never or hardly ever occurs. It is only when the nucleus pulposus has lost its normal characteristics—probably through poor nutrition subsequent to ischaemia, secondary to infection or trauma—that prolapse of the disc material takes place."

Major protrusions of disc material requiring surgery for their relief are uncommon in the young but by no means unheard of. The youngest in the author's practice was a girl of eleven seen in the early days of disc surgery, with clear evidence of a space occupying lesion. In this case, the protrusion was removed at operation by a well-known London neuro-surgeon, with complete relief of the sciatic scoliosis from which the girl had been suffering. It is difficult to believe that an otherwise normal child of this age can be suffering from idiopathic degeneration of the discs.

It is well known that there are no blood vessels in the nucleus of the disc nor in the annulus, save in its most superficial layers. There is, however, no suggestion that the disc material is not alive. The most accurate descriptions of the normal nuclear material suggest that it is made of mesenchymal cells in a three-dimensional lattice-work of fine collagen fibres covered with mucopolysaccharides and containing a high proportion of water.[20] As in any other part of the body, the living cells must be supplied with nourishment and must have their waste products removed in order to remain alive. The mechanism of nutrition of the disc is said to be by a colloid imbibition pump.[20, 21] Colloid substances have the property of attracting fluid which is known as the imbibition pressure. In the intervertebral disc, this tendency is balanced by the action of the hydraulic pressure which has the effect of trying to squeeze out fluid from the disc substance. When the disc imbibes fluid, its size increases, the fibres in the fibrocartilaginous annulus become taut and even if there were neither superincumbent weight nor muscle action, the imbibition process would reach a point of equilibrium. This is provided by the hydraulic pressure exerted on the disc substance by the end plates of the vertebral bodies above and below, and the fibrocartilage of the annulus around the sides. That the process of imbibition can continue is shown by the fact that when a horizontal section is made through a normal disc and the cut surface is then immersed in saline, the nuclear material swells and rises above the level of the surrounding annulus. When the patient sits down, or bends forwards, the hydrostatic pressure increases on the disc nucleus[8] and it is tempting to think that this increased pressure squeezes out fluid through the foramina in the vertebral end plate into the cancellous bone of the vertebral body. By virtue of the rich blood supply of this bone, metabolites are removed and nutrients are supplied to the tissue fluid. When the posture is changed to one in which the hydraulic pressure is lower, a fresh supply of fluid containing nutrients is sucked back by the imbibition pressure into the disc.

If this is the correct explanation of the process of disc nutrition, it is but a small step to assume that this imbibition pump is dependent for its function on mobility of the intervertebral joint at that level. When one considers the structure of the intervertebral joint as a whole and the pressures to which it is subjected, it is probably unreasonable to say that the loss of movement would be so complete as to prevent the pump working at all. On the other hand, it seems certain that the efficiency of such a pump would be interfered with by stiffness such that no movement is detectable on x-ray examination in flexion and extension. This loss of mobility in spinal joint injuries is established.

Thus it can be argued that the intervertebral joint stiffness secondary to injury may cause a defect in the nutrition of the disc. It is tempting to think that the observed disc degeneration in actual protrusions is due to this defect in nutrition. The suggestion that the loss of nutrition is partial rather than absolute could be part of the explanation for the delay so often observed between the original injury and the appearance of any sign of a true disc protrusion.

The theory that in spinal joint derangements the immediate source of pain arises in muscle is an attractive one in many ways. There must be very few people who have never experienced muscle pain from cramp. The chemical irritation of muscle by hypertonic saline is known to produce referred pain. The significant common factor in the wide variety of available treatments appears to be that they help to produce relaxation in muscle. Travell, Mennell and others have demonstrated particular patterns of pain arising from peripheral muscle. They have also shown that relief of the abnormal tension in the peripheral muscle results in abolition of the pain. It has been demonstrated that stimulation of deep muscles and other mesodermal tissue around the spinal joint will cause referred pain similar to clinical syndromes[5, 15, 16, 17, 22, 23]. In earlier editions the author postulated that the pain-producing contraction of muscle might in some way be abnormal and he likened this to modified cramp. Further work on the subject, particularly that by Korr,[25] does not support this theory. Korr's work, however, does give experimental evidence of overaction of the gamma system with abnormal spindle function in the muscles affected.

The concept of a muscle in which the resting length adjustment has been "turned up" to the maximum tightness appears to fit in well with clinical observations. The joint stiffness is rarely absolute. Movement away from the painful direction is nearly always possible but there remains a barrier to movement particularly in one direction. It seems reasonable to say that this is what would happen if muscle on one aspect of the joint were abnormally tight. The precise means by which the sensation of pain is produced is not clear. It is tempting to blame it on accumulation of pain-producing metabolites resulting from the overactivity which keeps the muscle tight. It is difficult, however, to accept that the circulation could be significantly compromised by the degree of tightness of muscle required to produce even the maximum shortening of its resting length. It may well be that the explanation will be found in an overflow of the continuing afferent impulses in the gamma system.

Wyke's work[24] referred to above did cause him to favour the metabolite theory for the production of the continuing pain.

REFERENCES

1 Froning, E. C. and Frohman, B. (1968), Motion of the lumbo-sacral spine after laminectomy and spine fusion, *J. Bone Jt. Surg.* **50**, 897–918.
2 Mixter, W. J. and Barr, J. S. (1934), Rupture of the intervertebral disc with involvement of the spinal canal, *New Engl. J. Med.* **211**, 210–215.
3 Charnley, J. (1958), Physical change in the prolapsed disc, *Lancet* **2**, 43–44.
4 Friberg, S. and Hult, L. (1951), Comparative study of abrodil myelogram and operative findings, *Acta orthopaed. scand.* **20**, 303–314.
5 Pedersen, H. E., Blunk, C. F. J. and Gardner, E. (1956), Anatomy of the lumbo-sacral posterior rami, *J. Bone Jt. Surg.* **38A**, 377–391.
6 Armstrong, J. R. (1965), *Lumbar Disc Lesions*, 3rd Ed., London, Livingstone.
7 Burke, G. L. (1964), *Backache from Occiput to Coccyx*, Vancouver, MacDonald.
8 Nachemson, A. and Morris, J. H. (1964), In vivo measurements of intradiscal pressure, *J. Bone Jt. Surg.* **46A**, 1077–1092.
9 Goldthwaite, G. (1911), The lumbo-sacral articulation, *Boston med. surg. J.* **164**, 365–372.
10 Gray, H. (1938), Sacro-iliac joint pain, *Int. Clin.* **2**, 54–96.
11 Cyriax, J. (1955), *Textbook of Orthopaedic Medicine*, London, Cassell.
12 Lindblom, K. (1951), Technique and results of diagnostic disc puncture and injection, *Acta orthopaed. scand.* **20**, 315–326.
13 Perey, O. (1951), Contrast medium examination of the intervertebral discs, *Acta orthopaed. scand.* **20**, 327–334.
14 Kellgren, J. H. (1949), Deep pain sensibility, *Lancet* **1**, 943–949.
15 Sinclair, D. C., Feindel, W. H., Weddell, G. and Falconer, M. A. (1948), The intervertebral ligaments as a source of referred pain. *J. Bone Jt. Surg.* **30B**, 514–521.
16 Feinstein, C., Langlin, J. N. K., Jameson, R. M. and Schiller, F. (1954), Experiments in pain referred from deep somatic structures, *J. Bone Jt. Surg.* **36A**, 981–997.
17 Hockaday, J. M. and Whitty, C. W. M. (1967), Patterns of referred pain in normal subjects, *Brain* **90**, 481–496.
18 Troup, J. D. G. (1968), Ph.D. Thesis, London University.
19 Roaf, R. (1958), Physical changes in the prolapsed disc, *Lancet* **2**, 265–266.
20 Sylven, B. (1951), On the biology of the nucleus pulposus, *Acta orthopaed. scand.* **20**, 275–279.

21 Hendry, N. G. C. (1958) The hydration of the nucleus pulposus, *J. Bone Jt. Surg.* **40B**, 132–144.

22 Kellgren, J. H. (1939), On the distribution of pain arising from deep somatic structures, *Clin. Sci.* **4**, 35–46.

23 Lewis, T. and Kellgren, J. H. (1939), Observations relating to referred pain, *Clin. Sci.* **4**, 47–71.

24 Wyke, B. (1970), The neurological basis of thoracic spinal pain, *Rheumatology and Physical Medicine* **10**, 356–366.

25 Korr, I. M. (1975), Proprioceptors and Somatic Dysfunction, *JAOA* **74**, 638–650.

12

The Scope of Manipulation

There is no doubt that lay manipulators have made claims which are as fatuous as they are fantastic. On the other hand, the medical profession itself must accept part of the responsibility for these claims. If a patient complains of pain in the chest, radiating down the left arm, associated with some shortness of breath and made worse by exercise, the obvious diagnosis is angina. Without very careful and repeated electrocardiography it may be extremely difficult to disprove this diagnosis. One of the most important differential diagnoses however, is a condition for which the treatment is very simple. This is a spinal joint lesion in the cervico-thoracic or T1–2 joints. A spinal joint lesion at this level can produce symptoms almost indistinguishable from an attack of angina.[1, 2] If such a patient with a doctor's diagnosis of angina visits and is cured by a lay manipulator, it is not unnatural that the manipulator will claim to have cured a case of angina. In this instance, the greater fault lies with the doctor who made the incorrect diagnosis; his fault is greater because his knowledge ought to embrace both possibilities and the means for distinguishing them. In this particular context, it is of interest to note that Lewis and Kellgren[3, 4] found that by injecting hypertonic saline to the left side of the spinous process of T1 they produced pain which was felt in the upper interscapular area, in the front of the upper chest and radiating down the inside of the left elbow and forearm with occasional skin tenderness on the ulnar aspect of the wrist. They further stated that in those with angina of effort, there was no difference in the symptoms produced by the injection from those of an actual attack of angina.

The association of gall-bladder disease with pain in the back of the chest is well known. The fact that a spinal joint lesion at the appropriate level (usually T7–8) can cause referred pain to the anterior abdominal wall and symptoms simulating those of gallbladder disease is not so well known. More than one such patient is described by MacDonald and Hargrave-Wilson.[5] If such a patient is diagnosed by a doctor as cholecystitis but is not cured, he or she may later visit a manipulator. If the manipulator then succeeds in relieving the symptoms, it is only reasonable for him to claim that he has cured a case of cholecystitis.

Unfortunately, the presence of long continued pain in a given segment tends to lead to chronic overaction of the muscles of that segment[6] and there is at least some evidence to suggest that in certain circumstances, this can result in the development of a joint lesion at that level sufficient to cause symptoms. In this event, the symptoms are likely to be similar to those which originally produced the excess tension in the muscle. In the case of chronic angina therefore, it is common to find excess muscle tension over a stiffened joint either at C7–T1 or T1–2 (see Appendix, Case 13).

The importance of this observation is that the finding of a joint lesion at that level does not exclude the possibility that the patient is also suffering from true angina. This likewise, applies to cholecystitis and to a wide variety of symptoms which can be produced by interference with nerve function through a spinal joint lesion or by some other totally different cause. It can be of great importance to recognise the possibility of the production of symptoms in this way and several cases showing the importance of this to the orthopaedic surgeon are given in the Appendix. Attention is drawn especially to hip pain as illustrated by Cases 10 and 11.

Lewis and Kellgren[3, 4] found that when they injected 6 per cent saline the referred pain appeared to be strictly segmental. This has not been confirmed by recent work in the same field.

Hockaday and Whitty[7] describe how the location of referred pain can be influenced by pre-existing pain in another segment. Feinstein et al.[8] describe subjects with pain reference to the frontal region from the 1st cervical segment.

These findings may explain why referred phenomena in clinical cases are sometimes associated with spinal joint lesions in segments other than the expected one.

The realisation that pain in almost any part of the body can be caused by spinal joint lesions is of course of enormous importance. Any orthopaedic surgeon practising in England has almost certainly had as one of his sessions, a County Council school children's orthopaedic clinic. Such clinics are made up of a relatively small variety of cases. The majority have flat feet, knock knees or bad posture. There is of course, the occasional scoliosis and the occasional congenital deformity. One of the most important subgroups is the children with painful feet. Experience of examining large numbers of children in this way soon makes one realise that while many of the painful feet are flat, there are very many more flat feet that are just as bad or worse, but which are totally painless. There are of course, the special classes with verrucae or with spasmodic flat feet, for both of which specific treatment is required.

There is also a not inconsiderable group of children with painful feet which are not flat. In other respects, the pain is no different from those with painful flat feet but without any other abnormality. Many of these children will say, if asked, that the pain tends to radiate up the leg when it is bad. In most it is worse after exercise but the pain is often particularly bad when all strain is off the legs when in bed at night. These observations led to the suspicion that the foot pain might be referred from a distant area and to the start of a systematic examination of the low back in all children complaining of foot pain without obvious cause. In this connection, flat foot was not accepted as a cause of pain in the absence of complications. The immediate and striking observation was of partial stiffness in the low lumbar spine. These findings appear to be universal in children with painful feet of this type. The equally remarkable observation is that they respond delightfully and rapidly to suitable treatment of the low back. After a few manipulations of the stiffened lumbar joints, the foot pain is much improved or has disappeared. These results compare very favourably with those of any form of treatment to the feet. It was found that after suitable low back treatment, the tone of the foot muscles often appeared to increase so that the feet were no longer flat enough to require treatment. This suggests that there is a motor as well as a sensory component in the nerve dysfunction. (Appendix, Cases 14 and 15.)

In discussing the origin of chiropractic, mention was made of Palmer's claim to have restored the hearing of a negro porter by manipulation of the upper thoracic spine. At first sight, this claim would appear to be completely contrary to anything known in anatomy, physiology or pathology. The claim, however, may not be quite as fantastic as it sounds, as is illustrated by one of the author's cases (Appendix, Case 16). The patient had no symptoms referable to the head or neck until after he had been injured when he gradually developed a Ménière's syndrome consisting of unilateral deafness, tinnitus and vertigo so severe that he almost always vomited, and the only relief he obtained was by going to bed. At first he was treated by manipulation of his stiffened neck joints and although this did help, the relief was transient and very far from complete. When the thoracic spine was examined, the lesion at the T4–5 joint was found and manipulative treatment to this joint resulted in dramatic and lasting relief of all symptoms referred to, including the deafness. The sympathetic supply to the vessels of the head and neck is said to arise from the T1 and 2 segments, with an occasional supply also from T3.[9] The dramatic improvement after treatment of the thoracic joint strongly suggests that this was the main source of the symptoms. Had the main source of the trouble been higher up, a temporary partial improvement might have occurred as the result of correction of tension at the lower level. In this patient the temporary partial improvement occurred when the higher levels were treated and the dramatic improvement only with treatment of the T4–5 joint. It may be that the anatomist's description of the sympathetic supply of the head and neck is incomplete or it may be that there are some other unknown factors.

Persistent pain following injury may also have a spinal origin. This can be seen following relatively simple injuries but it will be found from time to time in cases of fracture of an extremity and in these cases the pain usually comes as a somewhat unexpected development. It may begin soon after treatment has started, but when the pain should have subsided, or when treatment is nearly complete. A number of such cases are recorded in the Appendix, in particular Cases 17–23. Pain in these circumstances can take one of a variety of different forms. Commonly it is felt in or near the site of the distal injury although it may be more widespread than the original pain. This complication appears to be particularly common in injuries of the wrist caused by falling on the outstretched hand and in these the pain is commonly accompanied by swelling and stiffness of the fingers and hand. This syndrome is, of course, familiar to anyone who handles these fractures and in its more severe form it leads to stiffness requiring many months of treatment and often leaving permanent impairment. The author's observations strongly suggest that this syndrome is the result of spinal joint lesions and that the pain, swelling and other trophic disturbances apparently result from disordered nerve function resulting from these joint lesions. In some, the pain is felt also in the shoulder and in these, shoulder stiffness may also occur.

One can argue as to whether the spinal joint is injured in the trauma that caused the fracture or whether a pre-existing spinal joint lesion is reactivated as a result of the injury and its effects. In either case it is important to remember that the distal pain is likely to be referred to the site of the distal injury because there had previously been pain at that site, even if it is not in the same segment.[7] It is very unusual for these patients to have any pain or other symptoms in the neck and for this reason it is important to be on the alert for this complication. If a patient with a wrist injury presents with pain in excess of that expected or with stiffness and swelling of the fingers which is not immediately relieved by splitting the plaster, it is wise to examine the cervical spine without delay.

During the fifteen years that this was done in a busy accident practice, the author did not see any case of secondary trophic change in the wrist or hand except among patients who had initially been treated elsewhere and in whom the syndrome had been allowed to develop before the neck was treated.

These observations strongly suggest that the causative factor in the trophic changes of the wrist and hand is a disturbance of nerve function from trouble in the neck or upper back. If this complication is seen and recognised early, treatment of the neck or upper thoracic joint results in a rapid return to normal. If, however, the changes in the distal part have become advanced, they are not so easily reversed. It appears that as the result of nerve dysfunction a peripheral change takes place which is self-perpetuating. Even at this stage, treatment of the causative spinal joint trouble will often allow the distal condition to settle more rapidly. Treatment of the distal condition itself is however, usually required, and in some patients the causative spinal joint lesions may have resolved before the case comes to treatment.

Reflex sympathetic dystrophy was the term used by Evans[10] to describe distal changes occurring in association with injury. The term is used to include causalgia, bone atrophy, circulatory changes in the skin, sweating, oedema and other manifestations of what Evans calls "perversions" of the sympathetic nerve supply. The author's observation strongly suggests that faulty innervation caused by spinal joint lesions is one of the main factors in the production of this condition.

The most encouraging factor is that the condition appears to be rapidly reversible but only if treated early.

The recent work on axonal transport of proteins does appear to fit in with this concept of the causation of trophic changes. It will, however, be necessary to postulate that interference with normal nerve action by spinal somatic dysfunction can be sufficient to interrupt or alter the axoplasmic flow.

Unfortunately so far we appear to have no means of rapidly reversing the changes once they become established. When we know more about the precise nature of the proteins involved in both centripetal and centrifugal transport it may be possible to devise some means of replacing the missing factor in the periphery or even of removing an unwanted accumulation in the periphery due to failure of the centripetal mode. The clinical examples seen in the author's practice suggest that the phenomenon of trophic change is associated with disturbances in transport in either the sensorimotor or the autonomic fibres, or both.

Examples of a somewhat different syndrome are seen in Cases 24 and 25. In both of these, the treatment by immobilisation was completed and after this, there was the onset of pain more severe than had been experienced at the time of the injury. In Case 25 this was associated with severe cutaneous hyperalgesia, the picture being very like a true causalgia. In both cases, almost immediate relief followed manipulation and in Case 25 the manipulation was solely of a joint in the upper thoracic spine, suggesting that the effect was partly due to malfunction of the sympathetic as is found in causalgia.[11] Other examples of post-traumatic pain associated with spinal joint lesions are seen in Cases 7, 26, 27 and 28. These four are included specifically because in each case the symptoms were in patients awaiting settlement of a compensation claim, and in three the symptoms were somewhat indefinite and such as could easily have been dismissed as being due to a compensation neurosis. In all four cases there was marked improvement admitted before the claim was settled, which strongly suggests that the basis was physical, not neurotic.

In spinal injuries severe enough to cause vertebral compression fractures, strains sufficient to cause the production of symptoms are common in joints in the neighbourhood of the fracture. Two examples of this type of case are found in Appendix Cases 29 and 30. These two young men were injured in the same logging accident in British Columbia, both had fractured spines both were later seen and manipulated because of persistent lumbar pain. The relief of symptoms from the manipulative treatment was rapid and at least temporarily complete. Unfortunately, the alteration in spinal mechanics produced by the fracture appears to make it more likely for these patients to suffer recurrences needing further treatment but relief can be obtained by manipulation in the majority.

The question of pain transmission in sympathetic afferent nerves from the extremities is once again raised by the problem of explaining the relief obtained by the patient in Cases 31 and 32. In both these patients, the symptom in question was of pain in the leg. In both, relief ultimately came after treatment of joints in the thoracic region of the spine. In the one, the pain was causalgic in type and followed a compound fracture of the right tibia and fibula. In the other, the leg pain was a complication of low back trouble which had existed on and off for twenty years. Livingston[12] however discusses the evidence and concludes that no pain impulses from the extremities pass through the sympathetic chain.

Manipulative treatment at one level undoubtedly affects the muscle tension over neighbouring levels and this effect can apparently be found even at the far end of the spine from the level treated. In those in whom back trouble has been present for a number of years, it is common to find that there are stiffened joints at various levels. It may be quite difficult to discover which of these stiffened joints is the primary cause of the symptom for which the patient seeks relief. There may well be relief if a less important joint is treated, but it is likely to be partial and probably only temporary. This is apparently due to the alteration in muscle tension and spinal balance caused by correcting the lesion at the different level. If however, a primary joint is treated, one can expect the relief to be more complete and more lasting. Cases 31 and 32 have been included because in both of them the lumbar region of the spine had been treated on a number of occasions before the importance of the thoracic joints was discovered, but it was only when the thoracic spine was treated that relief was satisfactory. This strongly suggests that in both these cases it was the thoracic spine rather than the stiffened lumbar joints which was the cause of symptoms.

Livingston develops the concept that pain is not a primary sensation. This was first suggested by Weir Mitchell[13] and supported by Henry Head[14] and later by others. Pain sensation is regarded as the central result of recognition of a particular pattern of stimuli arriving at any one time. A mechanism is postulated by which incoming impulses are modified, both by the effect on their cord connections of impulses in other fibres, and by the reaction of the higher centres to impulses which arrived earlier in the fastest conducting fibres.

Melzack and Wall[15] in 1965 put forward a gate control theory of pain which proposes that perception of pain depends on three factors. First the intensity of the incoming stimulus. Secondly the modifying influence of the substantia gelatinosa which produces a negative feed-back from large fibre stimuli and a positive feed-back from stimuli arriving in the smaller fibres, and, thirdly, the modifying effect of centrifugal stimuli which themselves depend on the activity of the higher centres.

Melzack and Wall also agree that the theory that certain systems of fibres are specific for isolated sensory modalities is untenable and that the particular sensation produced depends on the pattern of the incoming impulses.

Livingston suggests that some of the anomalous pain seen in clinical practice is the result of what he terms a "persisting disorder of function" in the pool of internuncial neurones. He also describes paradoxical pain reference from trigger spots, especially in spinal muscles and remarks that "It serves to demonstrate ... that a peripherally situated trigger point is capable of initiating a pathologic state characterised by spreading reflexes, and probably dependent upon a disturbed physiologic status of the spinal centres."

It does not appear unreasonable to assume that the spinal origins of the sympathetic fibres to any part of an extremity have close connections with the spinal cord centres from which the somatic nerves to the part are distributed. The author's observations suggest that interference with function in the sympathetic nerves which supply the part can affect the "gate" mechanism which determines the perception of pain from that part, in spite of the difference in the spinal level of origin of the sympathetic and somatic nerves. These observations further suggest that a mechanical disturbance of function in the spinal joint can be one of the factors in the maintenance of Livingston's "disturbed physiologic status of the spinal centers."

The occurrence, as a result of spinal joint lesions, of distal self-perpetuating trophic changes could possibly help to explain a number of conditions, the origin of which is still uncertain. There is a striking similarity in the type and distribution of pain associated with a shoulder capsulitis with that found in certain types of brachial neuralgia due to spinal joint lesions. Indeed, many cases of shoulder capsulitis appear to start as a simple brachial neuralgia and to progress through a stage of pain in the shoulder muscles before the actual joint stiffness starts. If the neck and upper back are examined in any case of shoulder capsulitis, stiffness and muscle spasm will be found except perhaps in the very late stages. In the less usual case, in which shoulder adhesions have not developed, a dramatic increase in the range of movement can follow manipulative treatment to these joints. This improvement appears to be due to a relaxation of painful spasm in the muscles around the shoulder joint itself. Unfortunately, most cases are seen after adhesions have developed and at this stage the results of spinal joint treatment are no longer dramatic. Treatment of the spinal joints will have no effect on the adhesions but, if the spinal joints are still of themselves causing symptoms, these symptoms can be improved by such treatment.

When the symptom-producing spinal joints, and the associated areas of muscle spasm, have been treated adequately, it is usual to find that the pain in the shoulder begins to improve. With this relief of pain many patients start to recover movement in the shoulder. Such improvement may be quite rapid without any additional treatment. In those who do not recover their movement spontaneously, orthodox methods of mobilising the shoulder joint will be necessary, but if the pain has been relieved, the danger of producing an exacerbation is vastly less.

The carpal tunnel syndrome is probably another example of a symptom complex started by spinal joint lesions and maintained by local change caused by the secondary trophic disturbance.

The osteopaths long ago suggested that the "tennis elbow" might be a similar condition. The sympathetic supply to the elbow is said to arise from the 6th thoracic segment but this can probably vary one up or down in certain people. A spinal joint lesion in this neighbourhood is a common accompaniment of the tennis elbow although there rarely appears to be any complaint referable to the mid-thoracic spine. The author's experience with such cases certainly suggests that painful lesions in the elbow can be associated with thoracic joint disturbances at this level, although in the typical tennis elbow the local lesion also requires treatment.

The painful heel is probably another condition initiated by a spinal joint derangement and maintained by local changes. Although it can be associated with calcaneal spur formation, careful examination of a large series of x-rays of the heels will show that there are a similar proportion with and without spur formation among those who have no pain and among those who have pain. This strongly suggests that the spur has nothing to do with the symptoms. Appendix Case 8 is such a case which responded delightfully to sacro-iliac manipulation but unfortunately, this is not always found, some apparently failing to respond at all, even when there is firm evidence of a spinal joint lesion.

Cases 33, 34 and 35 are included as further examples of pain in the area of a distal lesion but which appeared to arise more in a spinal joint than in the local abnormality. Case 35 was a particularly striking example of relief which was most unexpected both to the author and to the general practitioner who referred the patient.

It was pointed out in an earlier chapter that when symptoms are complained of, the finding of a spinal joint lesion at the appropriate level does not excuse the doctor from a proper examination to exclude other possible causes. Some of the cases quoted suggest that even when there is a local lesion which appears to be sufficient cause, it may be wise to examine the spine at the level of emergence of the nerves to the part to exclude a spinal lesion as a cause of some of the symptoms.

Osteoarthritis of the hip is an example of a local lesion which is nearly always associated with a disturbance of spinal joint function. When we see x-rays showing severe osteoarthritis of the hip, we have a very natural tendency to explain to the patient what has happened to the hip joint and to assume that these changes are the cause of the pain. It appears that this is not always correct. Case 10 suggests that the spine was probably a major cause of the pain even before surgery. Case 38 is even more striking.

Age is not important of itself. Many octogenarians have been treated (gently) and obtained great relief. The youngest treated by the author was twenty-one months old (Case 36).

Collings[16] wrote, "If the neck is not a primary cause of pain, it may well be a secondary one, and if it is neglected therapeutically, the secondary cause may replace the primary, and an eminently curable condition is left uncured."

James Mennell[17] gave very similar advice in different words ". . . when ordinary medical remedies fail to bring about relief of symptoms, it is wise to consider the distribution of the nerves which supply the area or organ involved and then to examine the back in the neighbourhood of the origin of the appropriate nerve trunks."

REFERENCES

1 Annotation (1947), *Lancet* **1**, 685.
2 Josey, A. I. and Murphy, F. (1946), Ruptured intervertebral disc simulating angina pectoris, *J. Amer. med. Ass.* **131**, 581–587.
3 Lewis, T. and Kellgren, J. H. (1939), Observations relating to referred pain, *Cl. Sci.* **4**, 47–71.
4 Kellgren, J. H. (1939), On the distribution of pain arising from deep somatic structures, *Clin. Sci.* **4**, 35–46.
5 MacDonald, G. and Hargrave-Wilson, W. (1935), *The Osteopathic Lesion*, London, Heinemann.
6 Kellgren, J. H. (1949), Deep pain sensibility, *Lancet* **1**, 943–949.
7 Hockaday, J. H. and Whitty, C. W. M. (1967), Patterns of referred pain in normal subjects, *Brain* **90**, 481–496.
8 Feinstein, C., Langton, J. N. K., Jameson, R. M. and Schiller, F. (1954), Experiments in pain referred from deep somatic structures, *J. Bone Jt. Surg.* **36**, 981–997.
9 Mitchell, G. (1953), *The Anatomy of the Autonomic Nervous System*, Edinburgh, Livingstone.
10 Evans, J. A. (1946), Reflex sympathetic dystrophy, *Surg. Gynec. Obstet*, **82**, 36–43.
11 Barnes, R. (1954), Causalgia in "Perrpheral Nerve Injuries", M.R.C. Special Reports Series, 282, London, H.M.S.O.
12 Livingston, W. K. (1943), *Pain Mechanisms*, New York, Macmillan.
13 Mitchell, S. W. (1872), *Injuries to Nerves and Their Consequences*, Philadelphia, Lippincott.
14 Head, H. (1920), *Studies in Neurology*, London, Oxford University Press.
15 Melzack, R. and Wall, P. D. (1965), Pain Mechanisms. A New Theory, *Science* **150**, 971–979.
16 Collings, J. S. (1960), Techniques of manipulation, *Med. J. Aust.* **47**, (2) 55–60.
17 Mennell, J. B., *Physical Treatment by Movement and Massage*, 5th Ed. London, Churchill.

Appendix

CASE 1

Female, aged 34, housewife. Referred because of low back pain for four years on and off, with an acute attack for two weeks. She gave a history of having had a below-knee amputation of the right leg ten years before.

Examination showed that she was standing with the pelvis tilted upwards on the right and that the excess length of the right leg was enough to matter.

X-rays were taken with her weight bearing in the limb and these showed that the right hip joint was one inch higher than the left.

Examination confirmed the presence of the expected right sacro-iliac strain.

The patient was seen on seven occasions, on each of which the right sacro-iliac joint was treated by manipulation. There was little change as a result of the first treatment but marked relief following the second and subsequent treatments. When last seen, the leg length had been adjusted and her condition was very much improved.

CASE 2

Male, aged 28, fitter. Seen at the fracture clinic five days after a 16-ft fall.

He was complaining of severe pain in the left heel and calf but x-rays of the lower limb were normal.

Examination of the calf revealed no abnormality other than tenderness.

Examination of the low back showed an acute sacro-iliac strain and he required one manipulative treatment of this joint for complete relief. There had been no complaint of back pain.

CASE 3

Schoolgirl, aged 7. Seen at the fracture clinic ten days after she had jumped off a shed about 8 ft in height.

She complained of being unable to bear her weight on her left heel.

X-rays were normal and there was no clinical abnormality.

Examination of the low back showed a sacro-iliac strain which required two manipulations before relief was complete. There had been no complaint of back pain.

CASE 4

Female, aged 45, housewife. Complained of soreness in the front of the left knee with a history that she had fallen on to the knee some four months before.

There was no complaint of back pain at any time.

Examination did not reveal any abnormality in the knee joint other than some hyperalgesia of the skin over the patella.

Two manipulations of the left sacro-iliac joint relieved the symptoms completely.

CASE 5

Schoolgirl, aged 13. Complained of pain on the front of the patella and gave a history of having fallen on to that knee two weeks before.

There was no history of any back trouble nor of any complaint of back pain.

No abnormality was found in the knee other than a small, very tender nodule in the region of the pre-patellar bursa.

One manipulation of the sacro-iliac joint apparently relieved the symptoms completely. Two months later a recurrence caused by a second fall required one further treatment.

CASE 6

Schoolgirl, aged 11. Was seen at the fracture clinic six days after a fall on to the left knee over a vaulting horse at school.

She was complaining of pain in the knee and of inability to straighten the joint. Other than this limitation of extension there was no clinical abnormality in the knee and x-rays were normal.

Examination of the low back, however, revealed an acute strain of the sacro-iliac joint which required only one treatment for complete relief. There was no complaint of pain in the back.

CASE 7

Male, aged 46, factory cleaner. Seen for a medico-legal report following an industrial injury nine months previously, when he said that he had fallen on to his knee. He had had a great deal of pain in the knee followed by swelling of the leg and cramping in the calf and stiffness. The swelling and cramping had continued in spite of treatment initially by a plaster cylinder and then by a long course of physiotherapy.

A sacro-iliac strain was found during the course of the examination and it appeared likely to be at least a part cause of his symptoms. After a telephone conversation with his general practitioner he was manipulated at that joint and he later reported complete relief of the feeling of cramp in the calf although he continued to have some stiffness and swelling.

He was only seen on one occasion and the reported relief occurred before the compensation case was settled.

CASE 8

Male, aged 49, civil servant. Seen complaining of pain under the heel.

The examination showed no gross abnormality other than the tender spot commonly found. In this case it was under the medial calcaneal tuberosity.

X-rays did not show a spur.

Before coming to the clinic he had already received a course of physiotherapy and an injection of hydrocortisone into the painful area without relief.

Five manipulations of the sacro-iliac joint almost completely relieved his pain. There had been no complaint of pain in the back.

CASE 9

Female, aged 64, housewife. There was a long history of neck trouble for which she had had treatment by physiotherapy and for which she was wearing a collar and giving herself traction at home, with some relief.

Her complaints were of pain in the neck and headache.

She had stiffness at a number of levels in the neck and at first was treated by manipulation of joints in the mid and lower neck. She made only slight improvement.

At a later examination it became clear that the atlanto-occipital joint was more important than had at first been thought and as soon as this was treated she started to make a dramatic improvement. On her last seven visits during which she showed almost all the improvement, manipulative treatment was given to the atlanto-occipital joint alone.

When seen for low back trouble three and one half years later she had remained free from either headache or neck pain.

CASE 10

Male, aged 39, schoolteacher. Seen complaining of pain in the right hip.

He gave a history of injury in early adult life and had had increasing pain and lameness in the hip.

X-rays had shown early osteoarthritic changes and a Mc-Murray type osteotomy had been performed with plate fixation.

The improvement following the operation was less than expected and, after some months, the symptoms increased in spite of improvement in the x-ray pictures. The osteotomy was sound.

At this time examination of the low back showed clear evidence of strain, particularly at the L3–4 joint and he was treated by a manipulation of this joint on five occasions with very marked relief of pain. Six months later he returned for a further three treatments because of a recurrence. In the meantime he had returned to active sports.

CASE 11

Male, aged 17, student. Injured left hip at soccer in 1962 and complained of severe pain which originally affected the right hip also. It was thought at first that he had an early epiphyseal slip but x-rays continued to prove normal.

Unfortunately, in spite of extensive treatment including bed rest on traction, the pain persisted. He was seen by the author six years later when he had a full range of movement in the left hip but movement was painful, particularly rotation in flexion. All the x-rays were normal.

When the back was examined there was obvious stiffness and muscle spasm at the joint between lumbar 3 and 4. His pain was almost completely relieved by ten manipulative treatments but he had to return for further treatment after some months as the condition had recurred at sport. Relief was again obtained by manipulation.

CASE 12

Female, aged 38, housewife. Seen giving a long history of pain in the mid-thoracic region with a fresh attack of pain which had started three days before. The pain was associated with stiffness in the thoracic region and some radiation around the left ribs.

Examination showed that she had a spinal joint lesion at the

T7–8 joint and that associated with this, was an elevated 7th left rib.

Treatment of the spinal joint and costo-vertebral joints resulted in almost complete relief of pain after three treatments.

CASE 13

Male, aged 59, director. Complained of pain in the neck radiating to the chest and arm and pain in the low back. The original neck and low back pain had started seven years before and, three years before, the pain in the chest and left arm had started. This pain had been made much worse by exertion or by worry and had previously been diagnosed as angina.

Investigation, however, showed no abnormality on the electrocardiogram and manipulative treatment to the low cervical and upper thoracic spine relieved this pain almost completely. Other areas of the spine were also treated with relief.

The patient still finds it difficult to believe that his heart is normal. He has tended to suffer from recurrent pain in spite of treatment but the recurrences have so far always been relieved by further manipulative treatment.

CASE 14

Schoolboy, aged 11. Seen at a county council orthopaedic clinic with a complaint of pain under the heels which had been present for two years.

No abnormality was found locally.

Examination of the lumbar spine showed stiffness in the lower part and two manipulations apparently relieved the pain completely.

CASE 15

Male, aged 17, clerk. Complained of pain in the feet which had been present for some five years and he gave a history of having been seen at one of the county council clinics on many occasions with a diagnosis of flat feet.

Examination showed that the foot deformity was mild and apparently not sufficient to cause the pain.

Examination of the low back showed stiffness at two joints in the lumbar spine which were treated by manipulation on three occasions with almost complete relief of the pain in the feet. There was no complaint of pain in the back.

CASE 16

Male, aged 35, artificial inseminator. The history started when his head was driven downwards so that the neck was telescoped into the chest. At the time he had quite severe pain in the upper thoracic region and from then on it ached. About a month later he had the first of a long series of attacks typical of Ménière's syndrome which lasted for about 24 hr each. He had had a wide variety of investigations and treatment with no avail.

He was seen eighteen months after the accident at which time he had a number of stiff joints both in the neck and in the upper thoracic region. The importance of the thoracic region was not immediately appreciated but he did show distinct improvement, even after treatment of the cervical spine only. The improvement was much greater when the thoracic spine was treated and the joint which, to judge from the response to treatment, was the most important was that between the 4th and 5th thoracic vertebrae.

Unfortunately, he had to come a long way for treatment and he kept getting recurrences. He has now had the middle ear on the left side destroyed and although totally deaf on that side, he is free from attacks.

CASE 17

Male, aged 24, welder. First seen complaining of pain in the back of the carpus for eighteen months. He had had a long course of physiotherapy without relief. He gave a history that five years before he had hit his hand hard with a hammer at the same site.

Repeated x-rays had proved normal.

No radiation of pain was complained of but when the question was specifically put to him, he did say that the pain sometimes ran up the forearm.

Examination of the cervical spine showed an acute lesion and this was treated twice by manipulation with disappearance of symptoms. Six months later, he returned for one further treatment and he had remained free from symptoms when seen three years later for a fracture of the opposite wrist.

CASE 18

Female, aged 35, clerk. Seen at the fracture clinic for a crack fracture of the lower end of the radius which was treated by immobilisation in a plaster slab. Three days later she complained of severe pain in the thumb. The fracture was a minor one and there appeared to be no associated injury in the limb.

Examination of the neck, however, revealed an acute cervical lesion.

Treatment of this immediately lessened the pain. A second treatment was required one week later and two further treatments after removal of the plaster. She made a complete recovery without other treatment of any kind.

CASE 19

Male, aged 19, labourer. Sustained a fracture of the radial styloid process which was treated by immobilisation for five weeks in plaster.

When the plaster was removed he complained of pain in the ring and little fingers. There was no obvious local cause and the neck was examined. An acute cervical strain was found and treated once only by manipulation. He made a complete recovery without any other treatment.

CASE 20

Male, aged 28, unemployed at the time. Seen at the fracture clinic with a severe fracture of the lower end of the radius. This had been reduced and immobilised in plaster for nearly six weeks. Two weeks after removal of the plaster he returned complaining of severe pain in the wrist and of gross weakness of grip. There was no swelling and the wrist joint had an excellent range of movement.

Examination of the neck showed an acute lesion which was treated by manipulation on two occasions. Two years later he was seen again for a fracture of the opposite wrist and there had been no recurrence of the symptoms. He did not require any other form of treatment.

CASE 21

Female, aged 56, housewife. Seen at the fracture clinic for a crack fracture of the lower end of the radius which was treated by immobilisation in a plaster slab. Nine days after the fracture she complained of severe pain running from the wrist up the arm. There was no gross swelling and movements of the fingers were good.

A check x-ray proved satisfactory.

The neck was examined. A cervical joint lesion was found and treated by manipulation with relief of symptoms. This treatment was repeated two weeks after removal of the plaster because of some persistent soreness. No other treatment was needed.

CASE 22

Female, aged 62, housewife. Seen at the fracture clinic for a fracture of the base of the 5th metatarsal which was almost undisplaced and was treated by adhesive strapping only.

When seen two weeks later she complained of severe cramp all up the leg. At this time she also gave a history of old back trouble. The condition of the foot was satisfactory.

Examination of the low back showed a sacro-iliac strain which required two manipulative treatments for relief of the leg pain.

CASE 23

Male, aged 36, french polisher. Seen at the fracture clinic for fractures of the bases of the 2nd, 3rd and 4th metatarsals. This had been treated by a walking plaster for four weeks and thereafter he received a course of physiotherapy.

During this treatment, some seven weeks after removal of the plaster, he returned to the clinic complaining of pain in the foot, worse than at any time previously. Although the foot was still somewhat stiff and swollen, there did not appear to be any adequate cause for the pain and the lumbar spine was therefore examined.

A joint lesion was found and treated by manipulation. This gave almost complete relief in one treatment. There was no complaint of back pain.

CASE 24

Female, aged 53, housewife. Seen at the fracture clinic for a severe sprain of the wrist with a minor dorsal flake fracture. This was treated by immobilisation in plaster for five weeks.

When she returned after removal of the plaster she said that four days later she had started having severe pain in the hand with gross sweating and at the same time she got a headache.

No very obvious cause was found in the hand and examination of the neck showed an acute cervical joint lesion. The symptoms were completely relieved by two manipulations of the neck and she did not need any other treatment.

CASE 25

Schoolgirl, aged 13. Seen at the fracture clinic with a greenstick fracture of the left radius and ulna which had been satisfactorily reduced and immobilised in plaster. After three weeks, the plaster was removed and at first the result appeared to be very good. Six weeks after removal of the plaster, however, she returned complaining of very severe pain in the forearm which had started only two days before. The painful area was centred over the site of the fracture but spread for some distance in all directions and it was associated with gross hyperalgesia which made it almost impossible to handle the forearm at all.

A fresh x-ray showed sound union in excellent position.

Examination of the cervical spine did not show any gross abnormality. On looking lower down, however, there was an acute spinal joint lesion at the T4–5 level, although she did not make any complaint of the back.

One treatment of this joint (much to the surprise of both patient and her mother) gave relief within ten minutes and she did not have any recurrence of pain.

CASE 26

Male, aged 42, machine moulder. This man was seen for a medico-legal report five months after a crushing injury to the hand sustained in a press. The injury had caused very severe bruising but fortunately no major damage.

He had received one month's physiotherapy treatment with very little relief and complained of pain on gripping, weakness of the thumb and aching, particularly in the back of the wrist, extending up the forearm. The distribution of the pain suggested that it was at least partly due to a nerve irritation in the neck.

Examination of the cervical spine showed more than one joint strain.

After a consultation with the general practitioner these were treated on three occasions and the patient reported almost complete relief before the case came to trial.

CASE 27

Male, aged 60, stockman. Seen for medico-legal report following a road accident in which he had been knocked down by a motor-cycle and severely bruised. The injury had occurred six months before and he had received a course of twelve weeks' physiotherapy with only minor relief.

His complaint was of pain and stiffness in the right shoulder, sufficient to prevent him lifting anything heavy or even using his arm to chop sticks for the fire.

After consultation with the general practitioner, he was given three manipulative treatments to the neck and upper thoracic spine and within two months had returned to work.

A further report was requested and he was re-examined six months after the initial examination because the case had still not been settled. At that time he was still at work although he did find he needed to have lighter work than previously. He had not had any other treatment.

CASE 28

Male, aged 52, machinist. Seen for a medico-legal report complaining of weakness of grip and pain on using the right hand. This followed an injury when his right hand had been caught and badly twisted in a lathe. The only bone injury was a scaphoid fracture which had united soundly but the pain was such that he found it difficult even to turn a door knob with his right hand. He had, however, continued at work.

Again after consultation with his general practitioner, he was given a number of manipulative treatments to the cervical spine which resulted in marked lessening but not complete relief of the pain. When last seen, the case had still not been settled.

CASE 29

Male, aged 26, logger. First seen seven weeks after being struck in the back by a falling log. After striking him in the back the log had fallen on his right foot.

X-rays showed a crush fracture of the body of L4 and of the right cuboid.

He had been treated by rest in bed for his back and a walking plaster for the foot. Physiotherapy treatment was arranged for his back and foot and he improved satisfactorily but continued to have pain on bending, particularly when on strenuous exercises.

Four manipulative treatments to the L4–5 and lumbo-sacral joints resulted in complete relief of symptoms. In the meantime, the foot had settled completely on the physiotherapy treatment.

CASE 30

Male, aged 22, logger. First seen eleven weeks after being struck in the back by a log as a result of which he sustained a crush fracture of the 12th thoracic vertebra and an injury to the right knee.

X-rays of the knee were normal and a medial ligament tear was diagnosed. There was only very slight ligament laxity on examination.

He continued to complain of symptoms referred both to the back and the knee in spite of continuing physiotherapy and it was thought that he might also have torn the right medial meniscus.

Because of the continuing low back pain, the lower joints were examined and he was given three manipulative treatments to the right sacro-iliac joint, which resulted not only in apparent complete relief of the back pain, but also of the pain in the knee.

CASE 31

Male, aged 43, machinist. Sustained a compound fracture of the right tibia and fibula as the result of a heavy weight falling on the leg. The wound was small and clean and the fracture was treated by early excision of the wound, open reduction and internal fixation. From about the fourteenth post-operative day he complained of more pain than could be expected with the apparently satisfactory state of the fracture. The plaster had to be split and eventually removed except for a back shell, and he was grossly hyperalgesic on the front of the ankle and shin.

There was no neurological deficit although he did not like moving his foot at all because of the pain.

The fracture progressed to satisfactory union in the expected way and at no time was there any x-ray abnormality.

The extreme hyperalgesia remained and he was quite unable to bear weight for many months after union was complete.

At this stage the spinal column was examined in the hope of finding some possible cause for the over-sensitivity. As is the case in so many people, there was stiffness at a number of levels but no very gross muscle spasm. Subsequent examination, however, did indicate muscle spasm sufficient to be a cause of symptoms in the upper lumbar region and although he continued to complain of pain he was very much relieved by repeated manipulation of this area. He subsequently had the plate and screws removed. There was no gross abnormality and no sign of any inflammatory reaction. The condition does not appear to have been affected by the removal of the metal.

CASE 32

Male, aged 50, printer. Complaining of low back pain with radiation down the left leg to the foot. He gave a history of back pain having started following a strain during war service.

Examination at first suggested that the low lumbar region was basically responsible for his symptoms but although he improved a little with the first two manipulations, his condition thereafter remained static and disappointing until, at a more extensive re-examination, further lesions were found in the low thoracic region.

These required only three manipulative treatments to give him marked relief of both back and leg pain.

CASE 33

Male, aged 50, aeronautical engineer. Seen complaining of pain in the right knee which had originally started after kicking a ball awkwardly fifteen years before.

During the past twelve months the symptoms had been worse and he was getting pain even when he walked.

Examination showed a small cyst of the lateral meniscus but no other abnormality in the knee joint.

The low lumbar region was also examined and he was found to have a strain of the lumbo-sacral joint. The lumbo-sacral joint was treated by manipulation on four occasions with complete relief of pain. The cyst of the meniscus, of course, was unaltered but as it had not increased in size over a considerable period it was not felt necessary for it to be removed.

CASE 34

Male, aged 23, schoolmaster. Complained of a lump on the outer side of the right knee which had been present for three years and of pain in the knee on the outer side, but not always present.

Examination of the knee confirmed the presence of a cyst of the lateral meniscus and he was warned that this might require removal.

The nature of the pain prompted examination of the lumbar region and the pain was completely relieved at least temporarily by one treatment of the spinal joint strain.

CASE 35

Male, aged 75, retired coal miner. Seen giving a history of increasing pain and stiffness in both knees for about six years and, recently, pain radiating up both thighs.

Examination of the knees showed gross osteoarthritis with varus deformity due to loss of height of the medial tibial condyle on both sides. There was no abnormality in either hip joint but the radiation of pain up the thighs prompted the examination of the lumbar spine where it was found that he had well-marked stiffness with excess tension in the muscles suggesting that this was causing at least part of his symptoms.

It was decided to treat the lumbar spine first and much to the author's surprise, he improved so much in only three treatments that his knees had become very much more comfortable and he was once again able to go up and down stairs with comparative ease. He declined any further treatment although, of course, the basic condition of the knees was quite unchanged.

CASE 36

Female, aged 21 months. Seen at the fracture clinic because she was continuing to limp twelve days after a relatively minor fall in which she had apparently twisted her left foot.

There was no local abnormality and x-rays were normal.

Examination of the lumbar spine showed an acute strain which was treated by manipulation and this apparently relieved the symptoms completely.

CASE 37

Male, aged 29, car lease manager. Complained of back pain on and off for two years which had been started by a fall. A fresh attack had begun two months before and this time he also had right-sided sciatic pain. He had been in hospital for continuous traction for three weeks with partial relief and a myelogram showed a filling defect at the lumbo-sacral level on the right-side (Fig. 86).

Treatment of the right sacro-iliac joint resulted in almost immediate improvement in the severity of the pain, but the improvement in straight leg raising was slower. Over two months he was given a total of twelve treatments by manipulation and by the end of this was very much better. He returned after a further three months for two more treatments because of a mild recurrence of pain.

CASE 38

Male, age 56, salesman. Originally seen for pain in the upper back caused by a lifting strain. This responded very well to treatment by manipulation. Ten years later he returned complaining of pain in the low back for two weeks. Examination showed limitation of movement in the lumbar spine but he also had marked restriction of movement in the right hip joint. Flexion went to 90 degrees; in that position there was no rotation and the hip was in 5 degrees of fixed abduction. Examination of the

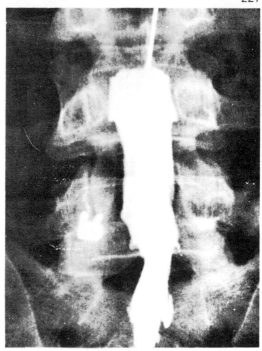

Fig. 86 Myelogram of
case 37 showing filling
defect on right side at
L5–S1.

individual joints in the lumbar spine showed limitation of movement at L3–4 with tight muscle on the right side. This joint
was treated by manipulation and he was given isometric exercises
for the adductor muscles of the right hip. Following the second
treatment he was very much better and was again able to reach
his toes and lace his shoe. The pain in the back and leg had almost
completely gone.

X-ray examination of the right hip showed severe osteoarthritis.

The interest of this case is that, had it not been for his previous
back trouble, it would have been easy to ascribe his symptoms to
the hip condition. The result of treatment indicates that the
lumbar spine was at least a major cause of the symptoms of
which he complained.

Index

Figures in bold type refer to illustrations